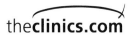

HEART FAILURE CLINICS

Diabetic-Hypertensive
Pre–Heart Failure Patient

GUEST EDITOR
David S.H. Bell, MB, FRCPEd, FRCPC

CONSULTING EDITORS
Jagat Narula, MD, PhD
James B. Young, MD

January 2006 • Volume 2 • Number 1

SAUNDERS

An Imprint of Elsevier, Inc.
PHILADELPHIA   LONDON   TORONTO   MONTREAL   SYDNEY   TOKYO

W.B. SAUNDERS COMPANY
A Division of Elsevier Inc.

1600 John F. Kennedy Boulevard • Suite 1800 • Philadelphia, Pennsylvania 19103-2899

http://www.theclinics.com

HEART FAILURE CLINICS	Volume 2, Number 1
January 2006	ISSN 1551-7136
Editor: Heather Cullen	ISBN 1-4160-3464-1

Reprints: For copies of 100 or more, of articles in this publication, please contact the Commercial Reprints Department, Elsevier Inc., 360 Park Avenue South, New York, New York 10010-1710. Tel.: (+1) 212-633-3813; Fax: (+1) 212-462-1935; e-mail: reprints@elsevier.com.

Heart Failure Clinics (ISSN 1551-7136) is published quarterly by W.B. Saunders, 360 Park Avenue South, New York, NY 10010-1710. Business and editorial offices: 1600 John F. Kennedy Boulevard, Suite 1800, Philadelphia, PA 19103-2899. Accounting and circulation offices: 6277 Sea Harbor Drive, Orlando, FL 32887-4800. Periodicals postage paid at New York, NY and additional mailing offices. Subscription prices are USD 145 per year for US individuals, USD 245 per year for US institutions, USD 50 per year for US students and residents, USD 175 per year for Canadian individuals, USD 275 per year for Canadian institutions, USD 175 per year for international individuals, USD 275 per year for international institutions and USD 60 per year for foreign students/residents. To receive student and resident rate, orders must be accompanied by name of affiliated institution, date of term, and the *signature* of program/residency coordinator on institution letterhead. Orders will be billed at individual rate until proof of status is received. Foreign air speed delivery is included in all *Clinics* subscription prices. All prices are subject to change without notice. POSTMASTER: Send address changes to *Heart Failure Clinics*, Elsevier Periodicals Customer Service, 6277 Sea Harbor Drive, Orlando, FL 32887-4800. **Customer Service: 1-800-654-2452 (US). From outside of the US, call (+1) 407-345-4000.**

Printed in the United States of America.

Cover artwork courtesy of Umberto M. Jezek.

CONSULTING EDITORS

JAGAT NARULA, MD, PhD, Professor, Medicine; Chief, Division of Cardiology; and Associate Dean, University of California Irvine School of Medicine, Irvine, California

JAMES B. YOUNG, MD, Chairman and Professor, Department of Medicine, Lerner College of Medicine; and George and Linda Kaufman Chair, Cleveland Clinic Foundation, Case Western Reserve University, Cleveland, Ohio

GUEST EDITOR

DAVID S.H. BELL, MB, FACP, FRCPEd, FRCPC, FACE, Birmingham, Alabama

CONTRIBUTORS

GEORGE L. BAKRIS, MD, Professor and Vice Chairman, Department of Preventive Medicine, Rush University Hypertension/Clinical Research Center, Department of Preventive Medicine, Rush University Medical Center, Chicago, Illinois

DAVID S.H. BELL, MB, FACP, FRCPEd, FRCPC, FACE, Birmingham, Alabama

ZVEZDANA BOGOJEVIC, MD, Research Coordinator, Rush University Hypertension/Clinical Research Center, Department of Preventive Medicine, Rush University Medical Center, Chicago, Illinois

CHRISTINA BRATCHER, MD, Assistant Professor of Medicine, Section of Endocrinology and Metabolism, Department of Medicine, Tulane University Health Sciences Center, New Orleans, Louisiana

KEVIN A. BYBEE, MD, Consulting Cardiologist, Assistant Clinical Professor, Department of Medicine, University of Missouri-Kansas City, Kansas City, Missouri

SAJAL DAS, MD, Research Fellow in Cardiovascular Disease, Mid America Heart Institute, Kansas City, Missouri

VIVIAN FONSECA, MD, Tullis Tulane Alumni Chair in Diabetes; Chief, Section of Endocrinology and Metabolism, Tulane University Health Sciences Center, New Orleans, Louisiana

MICHAEL B. FOWLER, MB, FRCP, Professor of Medicine, Division of Cardiovascular Medicine, Stanford University School of Medicine, Stanford, California

ALAN J. GARBER, MD, PhD, Professor of Medicine, Division of Endocrinology and Molecular and Cell Biology, Baylor College of Medicine, Houston, Texas

GURUSHANKAR GOVINDARAJAN, MD, Diabetes and Cardiovascular Disease Research Laboratory, Harry S. Truman Memorial Veterans Affairs Hospital, Columbia, Missouri

KHURSHID A. KHAN, MD, Post-Doctoral Endocrine Fellow, Cosmopolitan-International Endocrinology and Diabetes Center, Division of Endocrinology, Diabetes, and Metabolism, Department of Internal Medicine, University of Missouri–Columbia, Columbia, Missouri

MARY ANN LUKAS, MD, FACC, Senior Director, Cardiovascular Medicine Development Centre GlaxoSmithKline, Philadelphia, Pennsylvania

JAMES H. O'KEEFE, MD, Consulting Cardiologist, Clinical Professor, Department of Medicine, University of Missouri-Kansas City, Kansas City, Missouri

JAMES R. SOWERS, MD, FACE, FACP, FAHA, Thomas W. and Joan F. Burns Missouri Chair in Diabetology; Director, University of Missouri Diabetes and Cardiovascular Center; Associate Dean, Clinical Research; and Professor (Medicine, Physiology, and Pharmacology), Division of Nephrology, Department of Internal Medicine, University of Missouri–Columbia, Columbia, Missouri

TINA THETHI, MD, Fellow, Endocrinology, Metabolism, and Diabetes, Section of Endocrinology and Metabolism, Department of Medicine, Tulane University Health Sciences Center, New Orleans, Louisiana

ABU R. VASUDEVAN, MBBS, MD, MRCP(UK), Academic Instructor, Center for Cardiovascular Disease Prevention, Lipoprotein and Atherosclerosis Research Section, Baylor College of Medicine, Houston, Texas

T. BROOKS VAUGHAN, MD, Fellow, Division of Diabetes, Endocrinology, and Metabolism, University of Alabama at Birmingham, Birmingham, Alabama

ADAM WHALEY-CONNELL, DO, Post-Doctoral Fellow, Division of Nephrology, Department of Internal Medicine, University of Missouri–Columbia, Columbia, Missouri

RONALD M. WITTELES, MD, Fellow, Division of Cardiovascular Medicine, Stanford University School of Medicine, Stanford, California

KATHLEEN L. WYNE, MD, PhD, FACE, Assistant Professor, Division of Endocrinology and Metabolism, Department of Internal Medicine, University of Texas Southwestern Medical Center at Dallas, Dallas, Texas; Medical Director, St. Paul Diabetes Management Program, St. Paul University Hospital, St. Paul, Minnesota

CONTENTS

The association between the metabolic syndrome (MS) and congestive heart failure (CHF) has been less studied than the association of MS and coronary heart disease. Nevertheless, many facets of the syndrome can lead to CHF, and some emerging data point to a link between insulin resistance, inflammation, and CHF. Furthermore, medical treatment of CHF can affect insulin sensitivity, and treatment of the components of the MS may affect CHF. Further research is needed to elucidate these complex relationships so that we may develop more effective preventive and treatment strategies.

Up to half of the cases of heart failure are nonischemic in origin, and many of these patients are diagnosed with "idiopathic" dilated cardiomyopathy. Abundant evidence now demonstrates that insulin resistance is a primary etiologic factor for many of these cardiomyopathies. This article reviews the epidemiologic, clinical, and pathophysiologic evidence supporting this link.

Type 2 diabetes mellitus and hypertension, once considered different entities, are now recognized to share common etiologic mechanisms and outcomes. Renin-angiotensin-aldosterone system activation, insulin resistance, chronic low-grade inflammation, and oxidative stress collectively lead to endothelial dysfunction and subsequent atherosclerosis and cardiovascular disease. It is now possible to identify and intervene in high-risk populations, even before clinical diagnosis. Multidisciplinary management, including control of dietary patterns and increasing physical activity, as well as pharmaceutic management of hypertension and dyslipidemia, are necessary to reduce risk for cardiovascular disease and renal-disease-related events in patients who have diabetes mellitus.

Current evidence supports the idea that all patients who have diabetes mellitus be treated to reach the same lipid goals as patients who have coronary artery disease. The first priority for treating dyslipidemia in type 2 diabetes is to lower plasma levels of low-density lipoprotein cholesterol; the use of statins should be nearly universal in this population. Combination therapy is indicated for many patients who have diabetes to achieve target lipid goals. Ensuring good glycemic control and treating comorbid conditions, such as hypertension and obesity, according to established guidelines is vital. Using a comprehensive, multidisciplinary approach is key to diminishing morbidity and lowering mortality in individuals who have diabetes.

Chronic kidney disease (CKD) is a major public health concern; it is a cause and an effect of hypertension. Treatment of hypertension with agents that achieve blood pressure (BP) goals and reduce proteinuria helps prevent or slow the progression of nephropathy and reduce the incidence of cardiovascular events. The management of hypertension in CKD generally requires a minimum of three different and complementary antihypertensive medications, such as angiotensin-converting enzyme inhibitors, angiotensin receptor blockers, beta blockers, calcium channel blockers, diuretics, aldosterone antagonists, and vasodilators, to achieve a recommended BP goal of less than 130/80 mm Hg. Macroalbuminuria (proteinuria) and microalbuminurias should also be reduced as blood pressure is lowered toward the goal.

Therapy for diabetes, a multiorgan disease, must now treat the underlying disease process and not just lower the serum glucose level. Preventing vascular disease and progression to heart failure has become an important goal of therapy because of the epidemics of obesity and type 2 diabetes. Because type 2 diabetes mellitus is now being identified in youth and adolescents, heart failure will soon be seen in people in their third and fourth decades. Therapies to control blood glucose must now target the lipotoxicity and the inflammation and optimize the AMP-activated protein kinase system, in addition to lowering glucose levels, to prevent the epidemic of cardiac disease and heart failure that has been developing in recent years.

In years past, it was assumed that the association between diabetes and heart failure was largely based on the increased risk in the diabetic patient for ischemic heart disease. More recently, it has become evident that the relationship between these two diseases is more complex than was originally thought. The concept of a diabetic cardiomyopathy, independent of other known causes of cardiomyopathy (ischemic, hypertensive, alcoholic, or viral) has emerged as a potential explanation for this relationship. This article assesses the epidemiologic relationship between diabetes and cardiomyopathy and several major avenues of investigation into its pathophysiology.

Angiotensin-converting enzyme (ACE) inhibitors improve outcomes in patients who have congestive heart failure; however, not all patients are candidates for this therapy. Clinical trials show that angiotensin receptor blockers may be logical alternatives or adjuncts to ACE inhibitors for patients who cannot tolerate ACE inhibitor therapy, who have persistent symptoms despite otherwise optimal medical therapy, or to reduce the chances of additional hospital admissions for congestive heart failure.

The pathophysiologic effects of diabetes on the heart occur, in part, through activation of the sympathetic nervous system. To date, no randomized clinical trial has investigated beta blocker therapy prospectively in a population of patients who have diabetes and HF. The question of the efficacy of beta blockers in patients who have diabetes and HF and the concern over adverse metabolic effects has limited the use of these agents in this patient population. Clinical trial evidence and recent meta-analysis data confirm the efficacy of specific beta blockers in patients who have HF and diabetes. In addition, negative metabolic effects have not been seen with the use of the nonselective agent carvedilol. Therefore, in the absence of contraindications, beta blockade should not be withheld in treating patients who have diabetes and HF; and their use may be instrumental in preventing further progression of HF and death in this population.

FORTHCOMING ISSUES

RECENT ISSUES

HEART
FAILURE
CLINICS

ELSEVIER
SAUNDERS

Heart Failure Clin 2 (2006) xi – xii

Editorial

Heart Failure in Diabetes: *Are You Exhausted, Sweetheart?*

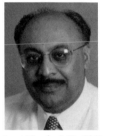 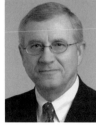

Jagat Narula, MD, PhD   James B. Young, MD
Consulting Editors

The number of patients who have type 2 diabetes is constantly rising and is predicted to exceed 200 million worldwide over the next decade. Even diabetic patients who have not previously experienced myocardial infarction have as high a risk of morbid cardiovascular events as non-diabetic patients who have previously experienced myocardial infarction. Diabetes is associated with a twofold to fivefold increase in the risk of heart failure (HF), independent of hypertension, body mass index, or coronary disease, and the risk is greater in women than in men. Nearly one third of patients who have heart failure and preserved left ventricular (LV) systolic function also have diabetes, and it is an important predictor of progression to overt HF in patients with asymptomatic LV systolic dysfunction. Furthermore, every 1% increase in hemoglobin A_{1c} level is associated with an increased risk of up to 16% for hospitalization for worsening HF or death, and approximately 30% of patients admitted to cardiac care units with heart failure have type 2 diabetes mellitus. In the ensuing decades, we will be faced with insurmountable demands on patient care, but we remain largely unprepared for the onslaught. Even more problematic is the definition of diabetic cardiomyopathy, and it is not clear whether diabetes plays an independent role in the pathogenesis of HF in the setting of diabetes mellitus.

It is believed that diabetes predisposes to LV dysfunction and HF by promoting atherogenic risk traits, obesity, LV hypertrophy, endothelial dysfunction, micro- and macrovascular coronary disease, and autonomic dysfunction. Even before these risk factors for cardiovascular disease come into play, metabolic alterations in diabetes exert independent effects on myocardium and vasculature. Altered substrate metabolism results in fatty acid over glucose use as the preferred pathway, which is associated with increased myocardial oxygen consumption and impaired mitochondrial homeostasis. These changes are accompanied eventually by the up-regulation of fetal gene programs and the down-regulation of reticular calcium uptake in cardiomyocytes. Furthermore, interstitial alterations caused by the accumulation of advanced glycosylation end products may contribute to ultrastructural and morphologic abnormalities in the myocardium and blood vessels that result in increased stiffness of the heart and diastolic cardiac dysfunction. A review of some of the recent literature [1] incriminates mitochondria in the pathogenesis of type 2 diabetes and heart failure, and it is likely that one may potentiate the other. Mutations in mtDNA and nuclear DNA genes encoding for mitochondrial metabolism have been reported in maternal diabetes, associated with deafness and maturity onset diabetes of the young. These subjects and affected family members demonstrate OXPHOS defects. Similarly, HF appears to be a manifestation of an enhanced level of mtDNA mutations and reactive oxygen species production and may reflect an accelerated phenomenon of ageing. Mutational studies have built causative links between mitochondrial energy metabolism, antioxidant gene expression, and HF. Oxidative mitochondrial stress is also well established as an inducer of apoptosis, which also constitutes an important pathologic substrate in HF. It seems advisable that the focus should shift to mitochondria in metabolic and degenerative diseases.

Given such an important role of diabetes in the evolution of heart failure, the American College of Cardiology-American Heart Association recommendations for diagnosis and management of heart failure classify patients who have diabetes (but no obvious myocardial structural abnormality) as stage A "pre-heart failure" patients and urge clinicians to try to prevent the development of overt or manifest LV systolic and diastolic dysfunction. Diabetes also contributes to asymptomatic, symptomatic, and more advanced stages of HF. This issue of *Heart Failure Clinics*, which is so brilliantly put together by Dr. Bell, is timely and focuses our attention on the pathogenesis of the diabetic affliction of the cardiovascular system, emphasizing the importance of the prevention of development of HF in diabetics.

Jagat Narula, MD, PhD
Professor, Medicine
Chief, Division of Cardiology
Associate Dean
University of California
School of Medicine
101 The City Drive
Building 53, Mail Route 81
Irvine, CA 92868-4080, USA
E-mail address: narula@uci.edu

James B. Young, MD
Chairman, Department of Medicine
Professor, Medicine
Lerner College of Medicine
Case Western Reserve University
Cleveland Clinic Foundation
9500 Euclid Avenue
Desk T-13
Cleveland, OH 44195, USA
E-mail address: young@ccf.org

Reference

[1] Wallace DC. A mitochondrial paradigm of metabolic and degenerative diseases, aging and cancer: a dawn for evolutionary medicine. Annu Rev Genet 2005;39: 359–407.

ELSEVIER
SAUNDERS

Heart Failure Clin 2 (2006) xiii – xvi

HEART
FAILURE
CLINICS

Preface

Diabetic-Hypertensive Pre–Heart Failure Patient

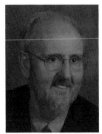

David S.H. Bell, MB, FRCPEd, FRCPC
Guest Editor

When I define type 2 diabetes as a cardiac condition manifesting as hyperglycemia, my endocrinology colleagues do not appreciate the definition. However, knowing that 75% of type 2 diabetic subjects will die of cardiovascular disease and two thirds of these subjects will die of cardiac disease justifies the definition [1].

A patient who has type 2 diabetes has as much chance of having a myocardial infarction as a non-diabetic patient who has already had one [2]. Because of this, type 2 diabetes has been classified as a cardiac equivalent, that is, the type 2 diabetic subject has at least a 20% chance of experiencing a cardiac event within the next decade. This places the type 2 diabetic patient in the same category as the patient who has peripheral vascular disease, cerebrovascular disease, or an abdominal aortic aneurysm because the actual risk for a cardiac event over 10 years in a type 2 diabetic patient is 36% [3]. Therefore, there is no such thing as primary prevention in the type 2 diabetic patient for whom the goals for controlling cardiac risk factors are those of secondary prevention.

When a type 2 diabetic patient has a myocardial infarction, the complication and mortality rates are twice as high as in a non-diabetic patient [4]. In fact, the most common cause of congestive heart failure after a myocardial infarction is the development of diabetes, and the best protection against developing heart failure is an exercise program that presumably decreases insulin resistance and the risk of heart failure [5].

However, if excessive prevalence and distribution of coronary artery disease were the only risk factors for cardiac events and mortality in the type 2 diabetic patient, then the risk of developing heart failure would not be as elevated. Seventy five percent of type 2 diabetic subjects are hypertensive, and this increased frequency of hypertension is associated with both hyperglycemia and insulin resistance [6]. Every molecule of glucose filtered and reabsorbed by the kidneys is accompanied by reabsorption of one molecule of sodium, which leads to salt and water retention [7]. Chronic hyperglycemia leads to glycosylation and cross-linking of proteins, premature ageing of collagen tissue, and premature stiffening of major arteries, leading to systolic hypertension, which is worsened by calcified atherosclerosis [6]. In addition, the high insulin level associated with insulin resistance, through insulin's action on the distal tubule of the kidney, increases both sodium retention and plasma volume [7,8]. High insulin levels also stimulate the sympathetic nervous system, which causes vasoconstriction, and hyperinsulinemia also up-regulates the AT1 receptor [9,10]. Because of the effects of hyperinsulinemia, 50% of non-diabetic hypertensive subjects are insulin resistant.

Although hypertension will lead to left ventricular hypertrophy, in the absence of hypertension, the

doi:10.1016/j.hfc.2006.01.006

heartfailure.theclinics.com

prevalence of left ventricular hypertrophy is increased in type 2 diabetic subjects. For example, in the Tayside study of a Scottish population [11] of newly diagnosed subjects who had type 2 diabetes, 32% of those without hypertension or coronary artery disease and who were not receiving an angiotensin-converting enzyme inhibitor were found by ECHO cardiography to have left ventricular hypertrophy. In a cross-sectional study of patients who had type 2 diabetes of varying duration, 71% were found to have left ventricular hypertrophy on ECHO cardiography [11]. It should be noted that, having left ventricular hypertrophy, at least in African Americans, is associated with a higher mortality rate (relative risk [RR] 2.4) than having left ventricular systolic dysfunction (RR 2.0) or extensive coronary artery disease (RR 1.6) [12,13].

While in the ECHO laboratory, if in these type 2 diabetic subjects we were to look for diastolic dysfunction by a sophisticated method such as tissue Doppler, we would find that 50% to 60% of these asymptomatic diabetic subjects had diastolic dysfunction. In Olmstead County, Minnesota, the prevalence of diastolic dysfunction in asymptomatic type 2 diabetic patients was found to be 52%, whereas in Quebec, Canada, it was 60% in a similar group [14,15]. Diastolic dysfunction is predicted by only two risk factors, elevated HbA_{1c} levels, and microalbuminuria [16,17]. Chronic hyperglycemia by glycosylating proteins causes cross-linking of collagen, which in turn increases myocardial fibrosis. Myocardial fibrosis is associated with microalbuminuria because microalbuminuria is a marker of endothelial dysfunction, which, in the myocardium, leads to multiple reperfusion injuries and fibrosis. The increased collagen content of the myocardium, resulting from both chronic hyperglycemia and endothelial dysfunction, stiffens the myocardium, leading to diastolic dysfunction, which is the principle characteristic of diabetic cardiomyopathy [17].

Thus, the subclinical ventricular dysfunction associated with diabetic cardiomyopathy becomes clinically apparent when hypertension and left ventricular hypertrophy are added to the diastolic dysfunction of diabetic cardiomyopathy, and with the addition of myocardial damage caused by coronary artery disease, ventricular failure occurs [18]. This "cardiotoxic triad" of diabetic cardiomyopathy, hypertension with left ventricular hypertrophy, and coronary artery disease leads to ventricular dysfunction, which in turn stimulates the renin-angiotensin and sympathetic nervous systems, leading to further injury to the myocardium, more ventricular hypertrophy, loss of cardiomyocytes to apoptosis, further increases in

ventricular fibrosis, and worsening left ventricular dysfunction. If left untreated, this condition of myocardial remodeling and increased stimulation of the renin-angiotensin and sympathetic nervous system leads to arrhythmia, pump failure, and death [19]. Therefore, therapies that reverse the stimulation of the renin-angiotensin and sympathetic nervous systems are crucial in preventing and reversing the process of myocardial remodeling, which results from the stimulation of these systems [19].

Based on the effects of type 2 diabetes on the myocardium and coronary arteries outlined above, it is not surprising that more than a third of type 2 diabetic patients die of heart failure and that 44% of heart failure patients admitted to hospitals in the United States have diabetes [20,21]. The high frequency of diabetes with heart failure is not only because diabetes leads to heart failure but also because heart failure leads to the development of diabetes. There is an increased prevalence of diabetes even in patients who have heart failure that is not caused by coronary artery disease, left ventricular hypertrophy, or diabetic cardiomyopathy. For example, a patient whose heart failure is caused by mechanical factors such as mitral incompetence has an increased risk of developing diabetes because of the high catecholamine levels that accompany ventricular dysfunction, leading to insulin resistance. If the pancreatic beta cells are not capable of producing enough insulin to overcome this increased insulin resistance then diabetes will develop. It has been shown clearly that the higher the New York Heart Association class of heart failure the higher is the prevalence of diabetes [22]. Thus, it is not surprising that the American Heart Association and the Heart Failure Society of America classify diabetes or hypertension as stage A heart failure. Stage A heart failure is defined as a high risk of heart failure that is not accompanied by structural heart disease or symptoms of heart failure [23].

In this edition of *Heart Failure Clinics*, we expand on the concept of diabetes and hypertension classified as stage A heart failure. The insulin resistance associated with the metabolic syndrome is not only associated with diabetes but also, even if diabetes never develops (as is the case in two thirds of insulin-resistant subjects), there is a twofold to fivefold increased risk of cardiovascular disease. This important concept is discussed in the first article by Drs. Theti, Bratcher, and Fonseca. Insulin resistance is also associated with a distinct cardiomyopathy, described in the second article by Drs. Witteles and Fowler. Insulin resistance leads to hypertension and dyslipidemia, both of which are worsened by the development of diabetes, and these risk factors are discussed in detail in articles three and four by Drs. Khan, Govindarajan, Whaley-Connell, and Sowers and Drs. Vasudevan and Garber, respectively.

Microalbuminuria can also be a manifestation of the insulin resistance syndrome, which as well as being a marker for future renal problems, is associated with endothelial dysfunction, atherosclerosis, and cardiac events. These concepts are discussed by Drs. Bogojevic and Bakris in the fifth article. All of the manifestations of insulin resistance syndrome (ie, hypertension, dyslipidemia, endothelial dysfunction, inflammation, platelet aggregation, and decreased fibrinolysis) can be worsened with the onset of diabetes and especially with uncontrolled hyperglycemia. The mechanisms for the cardiotoxic effects of hyperglycemia are discussed at length by Dr. Wynne in article six. Chronic hyperglycemia and microalbuminuria are the only known predictors of diabetic cardiomyopathy, and these and other manifestations and causes of diabetic cardiomyopathy are discussed by Drs. Vaughan and Bell in article seven. To avoid the development of heart failure and treat heart failure appropriately when it develops suppression of the renin-angiotensin and sympathetic nervous systems is essential. These topics are covered expertly by Drs. O'Keefe and Lucas in articles eight and nine, respectively.

It has been a rewarding challenge to edit this edition of *Heart Failure Clinics*, and I thank all of the authors who have contributed so much of their personal time to make this edition possible. The results of their efforts are both appreciated and worthwhile and will not only make the practicing cardiologist more aware of the cardiac manifestations of diabetes but also bring the specialties of cardiology and endocrinology and metabolism closer to the realization that we are all dealing with the same disease processes—insulin resistance and diabetes. Therefore, type 2 diabetes truly is a cardiac disease manifested by hyperglycemia.

David S.H. Bell, MB, FRCPEd, FRCPC
1020 26th Street South
Birmingham, AL 35205, USA
E-mail address: dshbell@yahoo.com

References

[1] Bell DSH. Drugs for cardiovascular risk reduction in the diabetic patient. Curr Diab Rep 2001;1:133–9.

[2] Haffner SM, Lehto S, Ronnemaa T, et al. Mortality from coronary heart disease in subjects with type 2 diabetes and in nondiabetic subjects with and without prior myocardial infarction. N Engl J Med 1998;339:229–34.

[3] Nutritional Cholesterol Education Program. National Heart, Lung and Blood Institute, National Institutes of Health; 1982. Bethesda, NHLBI, Publication no. NIH 02–5215.

[4] Miettinen H, Lehto S, Salomaa V, et al for the FINMONICA Myocardial Infarction Register Study Group. Impact of diabetes on mortality after the first myocardial infarction. Diabetes Care 1998;21:69–75.

[5] Lewis EF, Moye LA, Rouleau JL, et al. Predictors of late development of heart failure in stable survivors of myocardial infarction: the CARE study. J Am Coll Cardiol 2003;42:1446–53.

[6] Bell DSH. Hypertension in the person with diabetes. Am J Med Sci 1989;297:228–32.

[7] Wright EM. Renal Na(+)-glucose cotransporters. Am J Physiol Renal Physiol 2001;280:F10–8.

[8] Bell DSH. Understanding the role of insulin resistance for the treatment of diabetes and the reduction of cardiovascular risks. J Gend Specif Med 2002;5(Suppl 1):S1–14.

[9] Nielsen FS, Hansen HP, Jacobsen P, et al. Increased sympathetic activity during sleep and nocturnal hypertension in type 2 diabetic patients with diabetic nephropathy. Diabet Med 1999;16:555–62.

[10] Shinozaki K, Ayajiki K, Nishio Y, et al. Evidence for a causal role of the renin-angiotensin system in vascular dysfunction associated with insulin resistance. Hypertension 2004;43:255–62.

[11] Struthers AD, Morris AD. Screening for and treating left-ventricular abnormalities in diabetes mellitus: a new way of reducing cardiac deaths. Lancet 2002;359:1430–2.

[12] Dawson A, Morris AD, Struthers AD. The epidemiology of left ventricular hypertrophy in type 2 diabetes mellitus. Diabetologia 2005;48:1971–9.

[13] Liao Y, Cooper RS, McGee DL, et al. The relative effects of left ventricular hypertrophy, coronary artery disease, and ventricular dysfunction on survival among black adults. JAMA 1995;273:1592–7.

[14] Redfield MM, Jacobsen SJ, Burnett Jr JC, et al. Burden of systolic and diastolic ventricular dysfunction in the community: appreciating the scope of the heart failure epidemic. JAMA 2003;289:194–202.

[15] Poirier P, Bogaty P, Garneau C, et al. Diastolic dysfunction in normotensive men with well-controlled type 2 diabetes: importance of maneuvers in echocardiographic screening for preclinical diabetic cardiomyopathy. Diabetes Care 2001;24:5–10.

[16] Devereux RB, Roman MJ, Paranicas M, et al. Impact of diabetes on cardiac structure and function: the Strong Heart study. Circulation 2000;101:2271–6.

[17] Liu JE, Robbins DC, Palmieri V, et al. Association of albuminuria with systolic and diastolic left ventricular dysfunction in type 2 diabetes: the Strong Heart study. J Am Coll Cardiol 2003;42:2022–8.

[18] Bell DSH. Diabetic cardiomyopathy. Diabetes Care 2003;26:2949–51.

[19] Bell DSH. Heart failure: the frequent, forgotten, and often fatal complication of diabetes. Diabetes Care 2003;26:2433–41.

[20] Malmberg K, Ryden L, Hamsten A, et al for the Diabetes Insulin-Glucose in Acute Myocardial Infarction (DIGAMI) Study Group. Effects of insulin treatment on cause-specific one-year mortality and morbidity in diabetic patients with acute myocardial infarction. Eur Heart J 1996;17:1337–44.

[21] Adams Jr KF, Fonarow GC, Emerman CL, et al for the ADHERE Scientific Advisory Committee and Investigators. Characteristics and outcomes of patients hospitalized for heart failure in the United States: rationale, design, and preliminary observations from the first 100,000 cases in the Acute Decompensated Heart Failure National Registry (ADHERE). Am Heart J 2005;149(2):209–16.

[22] Tenenbaum A, Motro M, Fisman EZ, et al. Functional class in patients with heart failure is associated with the development of diabetes. Am J Med 2003; 114(4):271–5.

[23] Hunt SA, Abraham WT, Chin MH, et al for the ACC/AHA 2005 Guideline Update for the Diagnosis and Management of Chronic Heart Failure in the Adult–Summary Article. A report of the American College of Cardiology/American Heart Association task force on practice guidelines (Writing Committee to update the 2001 guidelines for the evaluation and management of heart failure): developed in collaboration with the American College of Chest Physicians and the International Society for Heart and Lung Transplantation: endorsed by the Heart Rhythm Society. Circulation 2005;112:1825–52.

Heart Failure Clin 2 (2006) 1 – 11

Metabolic Syndrome and Heart Failure

Tina Thethi, MD, Christina Bratcher, MD, Vivian Fonseca, MD*

Tulane University Health Sciences Center, New Orleans, LA, USA

The metabolic syndrome (MS) affects approximately one quarter of the population in developed countries [1]. Its presence is a major risk factor for development of both type 2 diabetes (T2DM) and atherosclerosis. The MS is a cluster of cardiovascular risk factors that are frequently associated with insulin resistance. Though it is synonymous with the "insulin resistance syndrome," not all patients who have the MS have insulin resistance [2]. The prevalence of cardiovascular disease (CVD) is two to three times higher in individuals who have the MS than in age-matched controls [1]. People who have the MS have a fivefold greater risk for developing T2DM. Early identification of subjects who have the MS is important, because they represent a target group for multiple life-style and pharmacologic interventions.

Because the MS leads to coronary artery disease (CAD), of which congestive heart failure (CHF) is a late-stage complication, the MS is likely to be an indirect but important primary cause of CHF. Few studies have explored the links between the MS and CHF. However, it is well recognized that obesity is associated with increased risk for CHF [3]. The purpose of this article is to highlight the known association between the MS and CHF and serve as an introduction to other articles in this issue that deal with the impact of treatment on MS-related CHF.

Prevalence

The global epidemic of T2DM is now well characterized [4]. However, data on the occurrence of the MS in populations are limited [5]. The lack of an internationally accepted definition has impeded epidemiologic work on the prevalence and antecedents of this syndrome [5]. Currently, the MS, a constellation of risk factors, is used to identify high-risk individuals beyond the traditional coronary risk factors, because of the association of the MS with subsequent development of CVD and diabetes [6–10]. Three definitions of the syndrome have been proposed, one by the World Health Organization (WHO), one by the US Third Report of the National Cholesterol Education Program, Adult Treatment Panel, 2001 (NCEP-ATP III), and one by the International Diabetes Federation (Box 1).

Data from the Third National Health and Nutrition Examination Survey (NHANES III) showed that, among United States adults aged 20 years or older, the MS is present in 23.8% of whites, 21.6% of blacks, and 31.9% of Hispanics. The NHANES III does not include data on American Indians [11,12]. Data from the Strong Heart Study (SHS), a longitudinal, population-based study of CVD and CVD risk factors, reveals that the prevalence of the MS in SHS men aged 45 to 49 years is 43.9%, compared with 20% among all men in NHANES III, a prevalence ratio of 2.18. The prevalence of the MS in SHS women in the same age group was 56.7%, compared with 23.1% among NHANES III women, a ratio of

---

Diabetes research and education at Tulane University Health Sciences Center is supported in part by the John C. Cudd Memorial Fund, the Tullis-Tulane Alumni Chair in Diabetes, and the Susan Harling Robinson Fellowship in Diabetes Research.

* Corresponding author. Section of Endocrinology and Metabolism, Department of Medicine, Tulane University Health Sciences Center, 1430 Tulane Avenue, SL-53, New Orleans, LA 70112.

E-mail address: vfonseca@tulane.edu (V. Fonseca).

Box 1. Current criteria for the diagnosis of the metabolic syndrome

World Health Organization

Diagnosis requires diagnosis of T2DM or impaired glucose tolerance (IGT) and any two of the following criteria. If glucose tolerance is normal, must demonstrate three other disorders.

- Current antihypertensive therapy and/or blood pressure >140/90
- Plasma triglycerides >1.7 mmol/L (150 mg/dL) and/or high-density lipoprotein <0.9 mmol/L (35 mg/dL) in men and <1.0 mmol/L (40 mg/dL) in women
- Body mass index >30 and/or waist/hip ratio >0.90 in men and >0.85 in women
- T2DM or IGT
- Microalbuminuria (ie, overnight urinary albumin excretion rate >20 mcg/min [30 mg/g creatinine].

US Third Report of the National Cholesterol Education Program, Adult Treatment Panel, 2001

Diagnosis requires any three of the following disorders:

- Blood pressure medication or blood pressure >130/85
- Plasma triglycerides >150 mg/dL, high-density lipoprotein cholesterol <40 mg/dL in men and <50 mg/dL in women
- Waist circumference >40 inches in men and >35 inches in women
- Fasting blood glucose >110 mg/dL (or >100 mg/dL)

International Diabetes Federation

Diagnosis requires central obesity plus any two of the other factors:

- Systolic blood pressure ≥130 or diastolic blood pressure ≥85 mm Hg, or treatment of previously diagnosed hypertension
- Raised triglycerides: >150 mg/dL (1.7 mmol/L), or specific treatment for this lipid abnormality or reduced high-density lipoprotein cholesterol: <40 mg/dL (1.03 mmol/L) in men and <50 mg/dL (1.29 mmol/L) in women or specific treatment for these lipid abnormalities[a]
- Central obesity (defined as waist circumference ≥94 cm for Europid men and ≥80 cm for Europid women, with ethnicity-specific values for other groups)
- Fasting plasma glucose ≥100 mg/dL (5.6 mmol/L) or previously diagnosed T2DM (If value is above 5.6 mmol/L or 100 mg/dL, an oral glucose tolerance test is strongly recommended but is not necessary to define presence of the syndrome.)

[a] Raised triglycerides and reduced high-density lipoprotein are considered two separate factors counting toward the two of four secondary factors necessary for diagnosis.

2.45. The ethnic differences in prevalence of the MS between SHS men and NHANES III men diminished with age, resulting in similar prevalences in the 60 to 69 and 70 to 74 age groups (~43% for SHS and NHANES III men in both age groups) [12]. However, in contrast to these similar prevalences among men in the older groups, the prevalence of the MS in SHS women was considerably higher than that in NHANES III women, even in the older participants. In the 60 to 69 and 70 to 74 age groups, the prevalence ratio contrasting SHS women to NHANES III women was 1.56. The overall prevalence of the MS was 55.2% in SHS participants aged 45 to 74 years [12]. These statistics emphasize the widespread prevalence of the MS and the importance of examining its causes and the available therapeutic options.

Insulin resistance

The insulin resistance syndrome overlaps considerably with the MS. It is a clustering of cardiovascular risk factors that are frequently, but not always, associated with obesity [13]. Although the underlying cause of the MS is a challenge to experts, it is believed that insulin resistance and central obesity are key factors in both the development of the cluster of risk factors and the long-term complications, such as CAD [14,15]. Attention was first drawn to the association of insulin resistance and obesity with T2DM, high plasma triglycerides, and low plasma high-density lipoprotein cholesterol [16,17]. Since that time, evidence has accumulated to support the association of this syndrome with CVD. Other cardiovascular risk factors that have been frequently included in the description of this syndrome are inflammation, abnormal fibrinolysis, and endothelial dysfunction [18]. It is unclear to what extent the components of this syndrome develop independently of one another or spring from "common soil" genetic abnormalities [19]. The increased prevalence of obesity and the frequent coexistence of these abnormalities in obese subjects have caused the syndrome to become a major clinical and public health concern [11].

Measurement of insulin resistance in epidemiologic studies is difficult, especially in patients who have advanced T2DM. Hyperinsulinemia is used to define insulin resistance in epidemiologic studies. Fasting plasma insulin alone or formulae based on plasma insulin and glucose (such as the homeostasis model assessment commonly known as HOMA) are used. Plasma insulin concentrations reflect both ambient glucose and pancreatic β-cell function (which decreases even before the onset of T2DM) [13]. Hence plasma insulin concentration is a poor marker of insulin resistance in subjects who have diabetes, although it remains useful in nondiabetic subjects. The nonstandardized nature of the insulin assay adds more difficulty to the interpretation of the levels. However, studies done using the clinical definitions have shown these subjects to be at increased risk for CVD.

Prospective studies suggest that hyperinsulinemia may be an important risk factor for ischemic heart disease [13]. The Quebec Heart Study studied men who were 45 to 76 years of age and who did not have ischemic heart disease [20]. A first ischemic event occurred in 114 men, who were then matched for age, body mass index, smoking habits, and alcohol consumption; a control was selected from among the 1989 men who remained free of ischemic heart disease during follow-up. Fasting insulin concentrations were higher by 18% in the case patients than in controls at baseline. High fasting plasma insulin concentrations were an independent predictor of ischemic heart disease, plasma triglycerides, and apo-

lipoprotein B, low-density lipoprotein cholesterol, and high-density lipoprotein cholesterol concentrations. High fasting plasma insulin concentration has also been associated with increased all-cause and cardiovascular mortality in Helsinki policemen independent of other risk factors [21]. However, it is important to realize that the relationship between insulin resistance and plasma insulin may not be linear [22].

The Uppsala Longitudinal Study of Adult Men [23] was a prospective, community-based observational study that investigated 1187 elderly (>70 years) men free from CHF and valvular heart disease at baseline between 1990 and 1995, with follow-up till 2002. This study examined variables reflecting insulin sensitivity (including euglycemic insulin clamp glucose disposal rate) and obesity, together with established risk factors for CHF, as predictors of subsequent incidence of CHF. In multivariate Cox proportional hazard models adjusted for established risk factors for CHF, increased risk for CHF was associated with a one-standard-deviation increase in the 2-hour glucose value of a glucose tolerance test, fasting serum proinsulin level, body mass index,

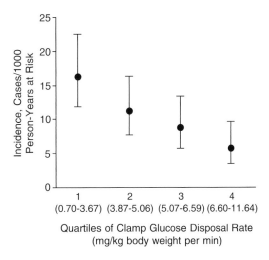

Fig. 1. Quartiles of clamp glucose disposal rate reflect insulin sensitivity. Error bars indicate 95% confidence intervals. In multivariate Cox proportional hazard models adjusted for established risk factors for CHF, increased risk for CHF was associated with a one-standard-deviation increase in the 2-hour glucose value of a glucose tolerance test, fasting serum proinsulin level, body mass index, and waist circumference. However, a one-standard-deviation increment in the clamp glucose disposal rate decreased the risk. (*From* Ingelsson E, Sundstrom J, Arnlov J, et al. Insulin resistance and risk of congestive heart failure. JAMA 2005;294(3):337; with permission.)

and waist circumference. However, a one-standard-deviation increment in the clamp glucose disposal rate decreased the risk (Fig. 1). Thus, in this study, insulin resistance predicted CHF incidence independent of established risk factors for CHF.

Proposed mechanisms linking insulin resistance with cardiovascular disease

The exact mechanism by which insulin resistance causes CVD is not known. However, insulin resistance is associated with several other cardiovascular risk factors, some of which are discussed in this section. Obesity is frequently associated with several of the components of the insulin resistance syndrome and may be critical for its development.

Moderate hyperglycemia

More than 17 million people in the United States currently have diabetes, and the number is rapidly increasing [24]. Randomized trials have clearly shown that decreasing the glycosylated hemoglobin level reduces this risk [25]. Multiple biochemical pathways are affected by the hyperglycemia of diabetes that could in the long term lead to CVD and CHF. However, few studies have examined this relationship, either in humans or in animals. The authors propose that the combination of insulin resistance and modest elevation of blood glucose (the term "dysglycemia" has been used in this context) also produces biochemical abnormalities that could lead to CVD.

Two studies have looked at the relationship between the levels of hemoglobin A1c and the risk for CVD. Khaw and colleagues [26] conducted a 6-year cohort study that analyzed the relationship of one hemoglobin A1c measurement to incident cardiovascular events in diabetic and nondiabetic men and women aged 45 to 79 years. After adjustment for systolic blood pressure, cholesterol level, body mass index, waist-to-hip ratio, smoking, and previous myocardial infarction or stroke, there was a 21% increase in cardiovascular events for every one percentage point increase in hemoglobin A1c level above 5% ($P < .001$). Similar relationships were observed for total mortality (22% for men [$P < .001$] and 28% for women [$P < .01$]) per one percentage point increase in hemoglobin A1c level. When both diabetes and actual hemoglobin A1c level were included in statistical models, only the hemoglobin A1c level (not diabetes) remained a significant predictor of incident cardiovascular events or death. This finding implies that a hemoglobin A1c level of 6.59% in a nondiabetic individual predicts a higher cardiovascular risk than a hemoglobin A1c level of 5.5% in a well-controlled diabetic individual. Thus, moderate hyperglycemia, such as that associated with the early stages of prediabetes, and impaired glucose tolerance are risk factors for CVD. These in turn are usually associated with insulin resistance.

Hypertension

It is well established that essential hypertension is frequently associated with insulin resistance. However, the impact of insulin resistance on blood pressure homeostasis is still a matter of debate. The association between hypertension and insulin resistance is more convincing in obese patients [13]. Multiple potential mechanisms by which insulin resistance may cause hypertension have been proposed [27]. These include resistance to insulin-mediated vasodilatation, impaired endothelial function, sympathetic nervous system overactivity, sodium retention, increased vascular sensitivity to the vasoconstrictor effect of pressor amines, and enhanced growth factor activity leading to proliferation of smooth muscle walls. Increased levels of aldosterone are found in the MS. A study by Kraus and colleagues [28] demonstrated that aldosterone directly affects major adipose functions, including stimulation of proinflammatory adipokines. Hypertension is itself a complex disorder with many causes, and not all patients who have essential hypertension are insulin resistant [13].

Obesity

Obesity alone is the cause of 11% of cases of cardiac failure in men and 14% of cases in women in the United States. The Framingham study showed that, after correction for other risk factors, for every point increase in body mass index, the risk for developing cardiac failure increased 5% in men and 7% in women [29]. Three pathophysiologic mechanisms explain the adverse effects of obesity on left ventricular function. First, there is an increase in ventricular preload secondary to increased plasma volume induced by the high fatty mass. Second, there is an increase in the left ventricular after-load due to the common association of hypertension generated by activation of the sympathetic nervous system by hyperinsulinism. Third, systolic and diastolic dysfunction result from changes in the myocardial genome, and CAD is induced by risk factors of atherosclerosis aggravated by obesity. The adipocyte also secretes a number of hormones that act directly or indirectly on the myocardium, namely angiotensin II, leptin, resistin, adrenomedulin, and cytokines [29].

Two forms of cardiac failure may be observed in obese patients. The more common is due to diastolic dysfunction [29]. In cases of cardiac failure due to obesity-related cardiomyopathy, loss of weight leads to improved functional status, a reduction of left ventricular remodeling, and an increase of the ejection fraction [29]. A study by Nasir and colleagues [30] assessed and compared the association of waist circumference and body mass index with the presence and severity of coronary artery calcium in 451 asymptomatic men free of known coronary heart disease. The subjects were divided into tertiles by waist circumference ($\leq$92 cm; 92.5–100 cm; $\geq$101 cm) and body mass index ($\leq$25.5 kg/m^2; 25.6–28.4 kg/m^2; $\geq$28.5 kg/m^2), respectively. The risk for coronary artery calcium was twofold higher among those men with a waist circumference in the highest tertile ($\geq$101 cm) compared with men with waist circumference of 92 cm or less. The relationship was found to be independent of body mass index, age, and conventional coronary heart disease risk factors. No significant association of body mass index with coronary artery calcium was observed. This study speaks of central obesity as being more strongly related to clinical and subclinical coronary heart disease endpoints than is body mass index. Another study by Santos and colleagues [31] reports higher levels of C-reactive protein (2.34 versus 1.36; $P < .001$) in patients who have the MS as compared with those who do not. The mean CRP levels were significantly higher in the presence of central obesity (2.45 versus 1.24; $P < .001$), high blood pressure (1.76 versus 1.12; $P < .001$), hypertriglyceridemia (2.17 versus 1.32; $P < .001$), and high fasting glucose (1.96 versus 1.46; $P = .032$). A significant increasing trend ($P < .001$) in the mean levels of CRP as the number of features of the MS increased was also found. The major features contributing to high CRP levels were central obesity and high blood pressure. In this study, the MS was defined by the Third Report of the Expert Panel on Detection, Evaluation, and Treatment of High Blood Cholesterol in Adults.

In a study by Wang and colleagues [32], obesity was also found to be an important, potentially modifiable risk factor for atrial fibrillation (AF). It was a prospective, community-based observational study involving a cohort of 5282 participants in Framingham who did not have baseline AF. During a mean follow-up of 13.7 years, 526 participants developed AF. The three categories of body mass index were <25, 25 to <30, and $\geq$ 30. Age-adjusted incidence rates

for AF were 9.7, 10.7, and 14.3 per 1000 person-years in men and 5.1, 8.6, and 9.9 per 1000 person-years in women. In multivariate analysis with adjustment for cardiovascular risk factors and interim myocardial infarction or heart failure, a 4% increase in AF risk per one-unit increment in body mass index was observed in men (95% confidence interval [CI], 1%–7%; $P = .02$) and a 4% increase was observed in women (95% CI, 1%–7%; $P = .009$). However, after adjustment for echocardiogram and atrial diameter, in addition to clinical risk factors, body mass index was no longer associated with AF risk. The relationship of AF with obesity is unclear, and further studies are needed to test this hypothesis and understand the mechanisms involved.

Dyslipidemia

Hyperlipidemia is well established as an equal risk factor in diabetics and nondiabetics. However, there are certain abnormalities in the lipoprotein pattern associated with insulin resistance that appear to convey risk and could be classified as nontraditional risk factors [13]. The hallmark of the "diabetic dyslipidemia" [33] is hypertriglyceridemia and low plasma high-density lipoprotein cholesterol concentration. In insulin-resistant patients, some qualitative changes in low-density lipoprotein (LDL) cholesterol result in "pattern B" distribution of LDL particles, consisting of smaller LDL particles that are more susceptible to oxidation and thus potentially more atherogenic [34]. At the level of the adipose tissue, insulin resistance may result in increased activity of hormone-sensitive lipase and therefore in increased breakdown of stored triglycerides. An increase in the circulating free fatty acids has also been proposed as having a causal role in the development of insulin resistance [35].

Inflammation

Inflammation has been associated with cardiovascular events in several studies. Low-grade inflammation may now be easily measured by the highly sensitive C-reactive protein (hs-CRP). Hence hs-CRP is an attractive risk marker in clinical practice [36–39]. Besides hs-CRP, several markers of inflammation have been used in various studies. Data suggest that plasma hs-CRP has a significant predictive value in determining the risk for future coronary events [37]. It is an acute-phase protein produced by the liver in response to production of cytokines such as interleukin 6 (IL-6), interleukin 1, and tumor necrosis factor-alpha (TNF-α). Fig. 2 summarizes the

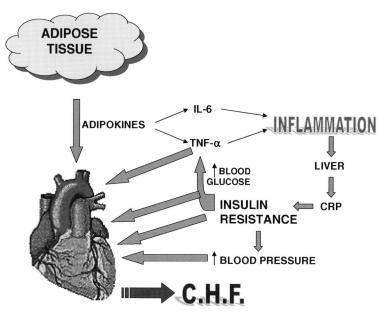

CHF=Congestive Heart Failure; IL-6=Interleukin-6; TNF-α=Tumor Necrosis Factor-alpha

Fig. 2. Adipose tissue is a source of adipokines, which may act directly on the heart. The adipokines may also cause the release of cytokines such as IL-6 and TNF-α, which, along with elevated blood pressure and blood glucose levels, also act on the heart. These parameters are increased in insulin resistance. Inflammation causes release of CRP from the liver, which also increases in insulin resistance. All these factors in obesity are hypothesized to have a link to CHF.

possible link between the cytokines and heart failure. Other inflammatory risk factors stimulate the production of IL-6, including oxidized lipids, infectious agents, and cytokine produced from adipocytes or other inflammatory cells. IL-6 in turn serves as a "messenger" cytokine that stimulates the production of CRP by the liver [36]. Several epidemiologic studies have documented that an elevated hs-CRP, is a good predictor [13] of the development of CAD, is a strong predictor of future coronary events in apparently healthy subjects and has prognostic value for acute coronary syndromes.

Many features of the MS are associated with increased levels of CRP. Hence it is important to evaluate the relationship between the two [40]. Among 14,719 apparently healthy women who were followed up for an 8-year period, 24% had the MS at entry into the study. At baseline, median CRP levels for those with zero, one, two, three, four, and five characteristics of the MS were 0.68, 1.09, 1.93, 3.01, 3.88, and 5.75 mg/L, respectively ($P < .0001$). Over the 8-year follow-up, cardiovascular event–free survival rates based on CRP levels above or below 3.0 mg/L were similar to survival rates based on

having three or more characteristics of the MS. At all levels of severity of the MS, however, CRP added prognostic information on subsequent risk [41]. The link between CRP and the MS could be substantially related to obesity and increased CRP production in response to the signal from adipose tissue through a variety of cytokines. An elevated CRP is common in patients with obesity; it was seen in 60% of women with a body mass index greater than 30 in one study [42].

In CHF patients, elevated plasma cytokine levels are associated with reduced functional status and adverse prognosis [43]. Plasma levels of TNF-α, an important mediator of inflammation, are elevated in people who have obesity and fall with weight loss [44]. A study by Vasan and colleagues [43] investigated the relationships of serum IL-6, CRP, and spontaneous TNF-α with CHF incidence among 732 elderly Framingham Study subjects (mean age 78 years, 67% women) who were free of prior myocardial infarction and CHF. The mean follow-up was 5.2 years, and 56 patients, 35 of whom were women, developed CHF. After adjustment for established risk factors, including the occurrence of myocardial infarction on follow-up, there was an increase in the risk for CHF per each tertile increment in cytokine production. It was 60% for TNF-α and 68% for IL-6 ($P = .04$ and .03, respectively, for the trend). A serum CRP level greater than or equal to 5 mg/dL was associated with a 2.8-fold increased risk of CHF ($P = .02$). Patients who had elevated levels of all three biomarkers had a markedly increased risk for CHF (hazards ratio 4.07; CI, 1.34–12.37; $P = .01$) compared with the other subjects.

Several studies have shown that circulating levels of TNF-α are elevated in patients who have advanced CHF. A study by Odeh and colleagues [45] examined the relationship between circulating TNF-α levels and severity of peripheral edema in patients with right heart failure. The values of circulating TNF-α levels (mean ± standard error of the mean) at presentation in the control group and in the right heart failure group, edema grades 0 to 3, were 2.98 ± 0.21, 4.22 ± 0.55, 4.67 ± 0.29, 7.66 ± 0.44, and 10.94 ± 0.67 pg/mL, respectively. There was a significant difference between the groups ($P < .0001$, analysis of variance), and a significant positive correlation was found between circulating TNF-α levels and severity of peripheral edema ($r = 0.77$; $P < .0001$). Serum TNF-α is an independent predictor of severity and mortality in stable pulmonary venous congestion [46].

Impaired fibrinolysis is now recognized as being an important component of the insulin resistance syndrome and probably contributes considerably to the increased risk for cardiovascular events [47,48]. Plasma plasminogen activator inhibitor (PAI)-1 antigen and activity are elevated in a wide variety of insulin-resistant patients, including obese patients with and without diabetes [13]. The greatest elevations in PAI-1 occur when there is a combination of hyperinsulinemia, hyperglycemia, and increased free fatty acids in obese, insulin-resistant patients [49]. Coagulation disorders also play a role in increasing the risk for coronary heart disease in patients who have T2DM. Many of the abnormalities are non-specific, and the association of insulin resistance with coagulation abnormalities is less robust than that with abnormal fibrinolysis [13]. In summary, increased PAI-1 and, to a lesser extent, increased coagulation are closely linked to insulin resistance and thereby could contribute to CVD. However, these abnormalities are probably less closely linked to CHF than are TNF and other inflammatory cytokines.

Microalbuminuria

Several studies have demonstrated that micro-albuminuria is a risk factor for cardiovascular events [50–54]. Recent data suggest that it may occur even in nondiabetics, may be a precursor of CVD, and may be related to insulin resistance [18,55–57]. In population-based studies, an increased urinary albumin excretion rate has been shown to cluster with other CVD risk factors, and it is included in the criteria used by the WHO to define the insulin resistance syndrome. Microalbuminuria has indeed been correlated with insulin levels (after an oral glucose load), salt sensitivity, resistance to insulin-mediated glucose uptake, central obesity, dyslipidemia, left ventricular hypertrophy, and the absence of nocturnal drops in both systolic and diastolic blood pressures [18].

Impact of various treatments on metabolic syndrome and risk for congestive heart failure

The concept of treating the insulin resistance syndrome in patients who have diabetes is well established [58]. In fact, because insulin resistance is associated with CVD, which is a major problem in clinical practice, clinicians treating patients who have diabetes have looked for ways to reduce cardiovascular risk beyond treating blood glucose, lipids, and hypertension [13,58]. A wide variety of pharmacologic agents may benefit patients with insulin resistance. These include insulin sensitizers like metformin and thiazolidinediones (TZDs), alpha glucosidase inhibitors, sulphonylureas, weight loss agents, and drugs that block the renin-angiotensin system.

Several therapeutic options are available for the treatment of heart failure. Besides pharmaceutical agents, life-style change plays a key role in the management of both CHF and the MS. In cases of obesity-related cardiomyopathy, loss of weight leads to an improved functional status, a reduction in left ventricular remodeling, and an increase in the ejection fraction [29,59]. A study done by LaMonte and colleagues [60] found significant inverse associations between fitness and MS incidence [13]. This study followed 1346 men and 56 women for a mean period of 5.7 years. After adjustment for potential confounders, multivariable hazard ratios for incident MS among men in the low, middle, and upper thirds of fitness were 1.0 (referent), 0.74 (95% CI, 0.65–0.84), and 0.47 (95% CI, 0.40–0.54) (linear trend $P < .001$). In women they were 1.0 (referent), 0.80 (95% CI, 0.44–1.46), and 0.37 (95% CI, 0.18–0.80) (linear trend $P = .01$), respectively.

The effect of TZDs on cardiovascular risk factors in people who have diabetes has been well studied. However, few studies have been conducted in patients who do not have diabetes. It has been demonstrated by Raji and colleagues [61] that rosiglitazone reduced 24-hour systolic blood pressure in some patients who had essential hypertension without diabetes. There was an inverse relationship between the change in systolic blood pressure and the change in insulin sensitivity. Thus, patients who had the greatest improvement in insulin sensitivity had the greatest reduction in blood pressure. This finding adds support to the concept that insulin resistance is associated with hypertension, and that this component in the pathophysiology of hypertension is treatable with insulin sensitization. TZDs have been shown to have many potentially beneficial effects on markers of inflammation in patients who have diabetes [13,62]. These effects have also been seen with other drugs used in clinical practice in patients who have diabetes and the MS. Both metformin and TZDs lower the level of the antifibrinolytic inflammatory cytokine PAI-1 [13]. Similarly, other markers of inflammation, such as hs-CRP and other important cytokines involved in inflammation and atherothrombosis, are reduced [13,62]. Nuclear factor κB (NFκB) activation is the key step in inflammation and may be involved in the process of early changes in the vasculature [63]. TZDs block activation and nuclear translocation of NFκB [64]. The effects of TZDs on inflammation have been primarily studied in patients who have T2DM. However, a study by Mohanty and colleagues [64] has demonstrated that rosiglitazone decreases a wide variety of markers of inflammation and causes a decrease in reactive oxygen species generation in obese nondiabetic patients. Endothelial function has been shown to be impaired in patients who have insulin resistance and diabetes. Studies have demonstrated that improvement in insulin sensitivity with TZDs improves vascular reactivity in the brachial artery in patients who have early diabetes, obese patients without diabetes, and women with polycystic ovary syndrome [64–67].

Good theoretic evidence supports the hypothesis that modulation of the renin- angiotensin system can improve insulin signaling. Angiotensin 2 interferes with insulin signaling at several sites in the pathway, and bradykinin, which is increased in patients treated with angiotensin converting enzyme inhibitors (ACEIs), enhances insulin signaling [68]. In addition, antiotensin receptor blockers (ARBs) have significant effects on markers of inflammation and have antioxidant properties [69–71].

As discussed earlier, metformin and TZDs are among the medications that improve insulin sensitivity. According to the prescribing information of the US Food and Drug Administration, metformin is contraindicated in patients who have heart failure

requiring drug therapy, and TZDS are not recommended for patients who have advanced heart failure [72]. The package insert for metformin says that the medication is contraindicated in diabetic patients receiving drug treatment for heart failure therapy, and TZDs are not recommended in diabetic patients with symptoms of advanced heart failure. Limited data suggest that metformin is often prescribed in patients with contraindications [72,73]. A serial cross-sectional measurement study using data from retrospective medical record abstraction was conducted by Masoudi and colleagues [72]. Two nationally representative samples of Medicare beneficiaries were examined who had been hospitalized with the primary diagnosis of heart failure and concomitant diabetes. In the 1998 to 1999 sample (n = 12,505), 7.1% of the patients were discharged with a prescription for metformin, 7.2% with a prescription for a TZD, and 13.5% with a prescription for either drug. In the 2000 to 2001 sample (n = 13,158), metformin use increased to 11.2%, TZD use to 16.1%, and use of either drug to 24.4% ($P < .001$ for all comparisons). Both metformin and TZDs exert positive effects on cardiovascular risk factors [72,74]. Yet these very drugs are either contraindicated or not recommended for use in heart failure.

In clinical trials, β-blocker therapy reduces morbidity and mortality in patients with CHF [75]. In heart failure patients, β-blockade may lower IL-6 levels, which may be related to improvement in left ventricular function [76]. β-blockers have also been shown to decrease cardiovascular risk in patients with hypertension and T2DM. However, some components of the MS are worsened by some β-blockers [75]. A randomized, double-blind, parallel-group trial (GEMINI) was conducted at 205 United States sites to compare the effects of carvedilol and metoprolol tartrate on glycemic control. Insulin sensitivity improved with carvedilol (−9.1%; $P = .004$) but not with metoprolol (−2.0%; $P = .48$); the between-group difference was −7.2% (95% CI, −13.8% to −0.2%). The effects of the two β-blockers on clinical outcomes need, however, to be compared in long-term clinical trials.

Summary

The association between the MS and CHF has been less studied than the association of MS and coronary heart disease. Nevertheless, many facets of the syndrome can lead to CHF, and some emerging data point to a link between insulin resistance, inflammation, and CHF. Furthermore, medical treatment of

CHF can affect insulin sensitivity, and treatment of the components of the MS may affect CHF. Further research is needed to elucidate these complex relationships so that we may develop more effective preventive and treatment strategies.

References

[1] Tkac I. Metabolic syndrome in relationship to type 2 diabetes and atherosclerosis. Diabetes Res Clin Pract 2005;68(Suppl 1):S2–9.

[2] Reynolds K, Muntner P, Fonseca V. Metabolic syndrome: underrated or underdiagnosed? Diabetes Care 2005;28:1831–2.

[3] Kenchaiah S, Evans JC, Levy D, et al. Obesity and the risk of heart failure. N Engl J Med 2002;347:305–13.

[4] Zimmet P, Alberti KG, Shaw J. Global and societal implications of the diabetes epidemic. Nature 2001; 414:782–7.

[5] Villegas R, Perry IJ, Creagh D, et al. Prevalence of the metabolic syndrome in middle-aged men and women. Diabetes Care 2003;26:3198–9.

[6] Alberti KG, Zimmet PZ. Definition, diagnosis and classification of diabetes mellitus and its complications. Part 1: diagnosis and classification of diabetes mellitus, provisional report of a WHO consultation. Diabet Med 1998;15:539–53.

[7] Laaksonen DE, Lakka HM, Niskanen LK, et al. Metabolic syndrome and development of diabetes mellitus: application and validation of recently suggested definitions of the metabolic syndrome in a prospective cohort study. Am J Epidemiol 2002;156: 1070–7.

[8] Lakka HM, Laaksonen DE, Lakka TA, et al. The metabolic syndrome and total and cardiovascular disease mortality in middle-aged men. JAMA 2002; 288:2709–16.

[9] Reaven GM. Banting lecture 1988. Role of insulin resistance in human disease. Diabetes 1988;37: 1595–607.

[10] Takamiya T, Zaky WR, Edmundowics D, et al. World Health Organization–defined metabolic syndrome is a better predictor of coronary calcium than the Adult Treatment Panel III criteria in American men aged 40–49 years. Diabetes Care 2004;27:2977–9.

[11] Ford ES, Giles WH, Dietz WH. Prevalence of the metabolic syndrome among US adults: findings from the third National Health and Nutrition Examination Survey. JAMA 2002;287:356–9.

[12] Resnick HE. Metabolic syndrome in American Indians. Diabetes Care 2002;25:1246–7.

[13] Fonseca V, Desouza C, Asnani S, et al. Nontraditional risk factors for cardiovascular disease in diabetes. Endocr Rev 2004;25:153–75.

[14] Buchanan TA, Xiang AH, Peters RK, et al. Preservation of pancreatic beta-cell function and prevention of type 2 diabetes by pharmacological treatment of insulin resistance in high-risk Hispanic women. Diabetes 2002;51:2796–803.

[15] Knowler WC, Barrett-Connor E, Fowler SE, et al. Reduction in the incidence of type 2 diabetes with lifestyle intervention or metformin. N Engl J Med 2002; 346:393–403.

[16] Reaven G. Metabolic syndrome: pathophysiology and implications for management of cardiovascular disease. Circulation 2002;106:286–8.

[17] Reaven GM. The role of insulin resistance and hyperinsulinemia in coronary heart disease. Metabolism 1992;41:16–9.

[18] Fonseca VA. Risk factors for coronary heart disease in diabetes. Ann Intern Med 2000;133:154–6.

[19] Stern MP. Diabetes and cardiovascular disease. The "common soil" hypothesis. Diabetes 1995;44: 369–74.

[20] Despres JP, Lamarche B, Mauriege P, et al. Hyperinsulinemia as an independent risk factor for ischemic heart disease. N Engl J Med 1996;334:952–7.

[21] Pyorala M, Miettinen H, Laakso M, et al. Plasma insulin and all-cause, cardiovascular, and noncardiovascular mortality: the 22-year follow-up results of the Helsinki Policemen Study. Diabetes Care 2000;23: 1097–102.

[22] Perry IJ, Wannamethee SG, Whincup PH, et al. Serum insulin and incident coronary heart disease in middle-aged British men. Am J Epidemiol 1996;144:224–34.

[23] Ingelsson E, Sundstrom J, Arnlov J, et al. Insulin resistance and risk of congestive heart failure. JAMA 2005;294:334–41.

[24] Harris MI, Flegal KM, Cowie CC, et al. Prevalence of diabetes, impaired fasting glucose, and impaired glucose tolerance in US adults. The Third National Health and Nutrition Examination Survey, 1988–1994. Diabetes Care 1998;21:518–24.

[25] Gerstein HC. Glycosylated hemoglobin: finally ready for prime time as a cardiovascular risk factor. Ann Intern Med 2004;141:475–6.

[26] Khaw KT, Wareham N, Bingham S, et al. Association of hemoglobin A1c with cardiovascular disease and mortality in adults: the European prospective investigation into cancer in Norfolk. Ann Intern Med 2004; 141:413–20.

[27] DeFronzo RA, Ferrannini E. Insulin resistance. A multifaceted syndrome responsible for NIDDM, obesity, hypertension, dyslipidemia, and atherosclerotic cardiovascular disease. Diabetes Care 1991;14:173–94.

[28] Kraus D, Jager J, Meier B, et al. Aldosterone inhibits uncoupling protein–1, induces insulin resistance, and stimulates proinflammatory adipokines in adipocytes. Horm Metab Res 2005;37:455–9.

[29] Galinier M, Pathak A, Roncalli J, et al. [Obesity and cardiac failure]. Arch Mal Coeur Vaiss 2005;98:39–45 [in French].

[30] Nasir K, Campbell CY, Santos RD, et al. The association of subclinical coronary atherosclerosis with abdominal and total obesity in asymptomatic men. Prev Cardiol 2005;8:143–8.

[31] Santos AC, Lopes C, Guimaraes JT, et al. Central obesity as a major determinant of increased high-sensitivity C-reactive protein in metabolic syndrome. Int J Obes (Lond) 2005;29(12):1452–6.

[32] Wang TJ, Parise H, Levy D, et al. Obesity and the risk of new-onset atrial fibrillation. JAMA 2004;292:2471–7.

[33] Sniderman AD, Scantlebury T, Cianflone K. Hypertriglyceridemic hyperapob: the unappreciated atherogenic dyslipoproteinemia in type 2 diabetes mellitus. Ann Intern Med 2001;135:447–59.

[34] Reaven GM, Chen YD, Jeppesen J, et al. Insulin resistance and hyperinsulinemia in individuals with small, dense low density lipoprotein particles. J Clin Invest 1993;92:141–6.

[35] Boden G, Lebed B, Schatz M, et al. Effects of acute changes of plasma free fatty acids on intramyocellular fat content and insulin resistance in healthy subjects. Diabetes 2001;50:1612–7.

[36] Jialal I, Devaraj S. Inflammation and atherosclerosis: the value of the high-sensitivity C-reactive protein assay as a risk marker. Am J Clin Pathol 2001;116(Suppl):S108–15.

[37] Ridker PM. Evaluating novel cardiovascular risk factors: can we better predict heart attacks? Ann Intern Med 1999;130:933–7.

[38] Ridker PM, Stampfer MJ, Rifai N. Novel risk factors for systemic atherosclerosis: a comparison of C-reactive protein, fibrinogen, homocysteine, lipoprotein(a), and standard cholesterol screening as predictors of peripheral arterial disease. JAMA 2001;285:2481–5.

[39] Rifai N, Ridker PM. High-sensitivity C-reactive protein: a novel and promising marker of coronary heart disease. Clin Chem 2001;47:403–11.

[40] Ford ES. The metabolic syndrome and C-reactive protein, fibrinogen, and leukocyte count: findings from the Third National Health and Nutrition Examination Survey. Atherosclerosis 2003;168:351–8.

[41] Ridker PM, Buring JE, Cook NR, et al. C-reactive protein, the metabolic syndrome, and risk of incident cardiovascular events: an 8-year follow-up of 14 719 initially healthy American women. Circulation 2003;107:391–7.

[42] Visser M, Bouter LM, McQuillan GM, et al. Elevated C-reactive protein levels in overweight and obese adults. JAMA 1999;282:2131–5.

[43] Vasan RS, Sullivan LM, Roubenoff R, et al. Inflammatory markers and risk of heart failure in elderly subjects without prior myocardial infarction: the Framingham Heart Study. Circulation 2003;107:1486–91.

[44] Dandona P, Weinstock R, Thusu K, et al. Tumor necrosis factor–alpha in sera of obese patients: fall with weight loss. J Clin Endocrinol Metab 1998;83:2907–10.

[45] Odeh M., Sabo E., Oliven A. Circulating levels of tumor necrosis factor – alpha correlate positively with severity of peripheral oedema in patients with right heart failure. Eur J Heart Fail 2005. Aug 18; epub ahead of print.

[46] Rodriguez-Reyna TS, Arrieta O, Castillo-Martinez L, et al. Tumour Necrosis Factor alpha and Troponin T as predictors of poor prognosis in patients with stable heart failure. Clin Invest Med 2005;28:23–9.

[47] Haffner SM, D'Agostino Jr R, Mykkanen L, et al. Insulin sensitivity in subjects with type 2 diabetes. Relationship to cardiovascular risk factors: the Insulin Resistance Atherosclerosis Study. Diabetes Care 1999;22:562–8.

[48] Sobel BE. Insulin resistance and thrombosis: a cardiologist's view. Am J Cardiol 1999;84:37J–41J.

[49] Calles-Escandon J, Mirza SA, Sobel BE, et al. Induction of hyperinsulinemia combined with hyperglycemia and hypertriglyceridemia increases plasminogen activator inhibitor 1 in blood in normal human subjects. Diabetes 1998;47:290–3.

[50] Deckert T, Kofoed-Enevoldsen A, Norgaard K, et al. Microalbuminuria. Implications for micro- and macrovascular disease. Diabetes Care 1992;15:1181–91.

[51] Gerstein HC, Mann JF, Yi Q, et al. Albuminuria and risk of cardiovascular events, death, and heart failure in diabetic and nondiabetic individuals. JAMA 2001;286:421–6.

[52] Spoelstra-de Man AM, Brouwer CB, Stehouwer CD, et al. Rapid progression of albumin excretion is an independent predictor of cardiovascular mortality in patients with type 2 diabetes and microalbuminuria. Diabetes Care 2001;24:2097–101.

[53] Tuttle KR, Puhlman ME, Cooney SK, et al. Urinary albumin and insulin as predictors of coronary artery disease: an angiographic study. Am J Kidney Dis 1999;34:918–25.

[54] Winocour PH, Harland JO, Millar JP, et al. Microalbuminuria and associated cardiovascular risk factors in the community. Atherosclerosis 1992;93:71–81.

[55] Pinkney JH, Denver AE, Mohamed-Ali V, et al. Insulin resistance in non–insulin-dependent diabetes mellitus is associated with microalbuminuria independently of ambulatory blood pressure. J Diabetes Complications 1995;9:230–3.

[56] Wasada T, Katsumori K, Saeki A, et al. Urinary albumin excretion rate is related to insulin resistance in normotensive subjects with impaired glucose tolerance. Diabetes Res Clin Pract 1997;34:157–62.

[57] Yudkin JS. Hyperinsulinaemia, insulin resistance, microalbuminuria and the risk of coronary heart disease. Ann Med 1996;28:433–8.

[58] Jawa AA, Fonseca VA. Role of insulin secretagogues and insulin sensitizing agents in the prevention of cardiovascular disease in patients who have diabetes. Cardiol Clin 2005;23:119–38.

[59] Alpert MA. Management of obesity cardiomyopathy. Am J Med Sci 2001;321:237–41.

[60] LaMonte MJ, Barlow CE, Jurca R, et al. Cardiorespiratory fitness is inversely associated with the incidence of metabolic syndrome: a prospective study of men and women. Circulation 2005;112:505–12.

[61] Raji A, Seely EW, Bekins SA, et al. Rosiglitazone improves insulin sensitivity and lowers blood pres-

sure in hypertensive patients. Diabetes Care 2003;26: 172–8.

[62] Haffner SM, Greenberg AS, Weston WM, et al. Effect of rosiglitazone treatment on nontraditional markers of cardiovascular disease in patients with type 2 diabetes mellitus. Circulation 2002;106:679–84.

[63] Shoelson SE, Lee J, Yuan M. Inflammation and the IKK beta/I kappa B/NF-kappa B axis in obesity- and diet-induced insulin resistance. Int J Obes Relat Metab Disord 2003;27(Suppl 3):S49–52.

[64] Mohanty P, Aljada A, Ghanim H, et al. Evidence for a potent antiinflammatory effect of rosiglitazone. J Clin Endocrinol Metab 2004;89:2728–35.

[65] Hetzel J, Balletshofer B, Rittig K, et al. Rapid effects of rosiglitazone treatment on endothelial function and inflammatory biomarkers. Arterioscler Thromb Vasc Biol 2005;25:1804–9.

[66] Tarkun I, Cetinarslan B, Turemen E, et al. Effect of rosiglitazone on insulin resistance, C-reactive protein and endothelial function in non-obese young women with polycystic ovary syndrome. Eur J Endocrinol 2005;153:115–21.

[67] Wang TD, Chen WJ, Lin JW, et al. Effects of rosiglitazone on endothelial function, C-reactive protein, and components of the metabolic syndrome in non-diabetic patients with the metabolic syndrome. Am J Cardiol 2004;93:362–5.

[68] Henriksen EJ, Jacob S. Modulation of metabolic control by angiotensin converting enzyme (ACE) inhibition. J Cell Physiol 2003;196:171–9.

[69] Khan BV, Navalkar S, Khan QA, et al. Irbesartan, an angiotensin type 1 receptor inhibitor, regulates the vascular oxidative state in patients with coronary artery disease. J Am Coll Cardiol 2001;38:1662–7.

[70] Navalkar S, Parthasarathy S, Santanam N, et al. Irbesartan, an angiotensin type 1 receptor inhibitor, regulates markers of inflammation in patients with premature atherosclerosis. J Am Coll Cardiol 2001; 37:440–4.

[71] Schieffer B, Bunte C, Witte J, et al. Comparative effects of AT1-antagonism and angiotensin-converting enzyme inhibition on markers of inflammation and platelet aggregation in patients with coronary artery disease. J Am Coll Cardiol 2004;44:362–8.

[72] Masoudi FA, Wang Y, Inzucchi SE, et al. Metformin and thiazolidinedione use in Medicare patients with heart failure. JAMA 2003;290:81–5.

[73] Horlen C, Malone R, Bryant B, et al. Frequency of inappropriate metformin prescriptions. JAMA 2002; 287:2504–5.

[74] Parulkar AA, Pendergrass ML, Granda-Ayala R, et al. Nonhypoglycemic effects of thiazolidinediones. Ann Intern Med 2001;134:61–71.

[75] Bakris GL, Fonseca V, Katholi RE, et al. Metabolic effects of carvedilol vs metoprolol in patients with type 2 diabetes mellitus and hypertension: a randomized controlled trial. JAMA 2004;292:2227–36.

[76] Mayer B, Holmer SR, Hengstenberg C, et al. Functional improvement in heart failure patients treated with beta-blockers is associated with a decline of cytokine levels. Int J Cardiol 2005;103:182–6.

ELSEVIER
SAUNDERS

Heart Failure Clin 2 (2006) 13 – 23

HEART
FAILURE
CLINICS

Cardiomyopathy of Insulin Resistance

Ronald M. Witteles, MD, Michael B. Fowler, MB, FRCP*

Stanford University School of Medicine, Stanford, CA, USA

For many patients diagnosed with heart failure, the underlying etiology remains elusive. Up to half of heart failure cases are not the result of coronary artery disease, and most of these are deemed "idiopathic" in origin. A further understanding of the cause of heart failure in these individuals could lead to great improvements in prevention and treatment of the disease. A review of insulin resistance and heart failure offers striking similarities. The two diseases are increasing in prevalence, paralleling the increase of obesity in society. Both states involve dysregulation of several neurohormonal systems – most notably the renin-angiotensin-aldosterone pathway, nitric oxide metabolism, and the sympathetic nervous system. Both states involve harmful upregulation of inflammatory mediators. Abundant epidemiologic, clinical, and basic science evidence now supports a primary causative role for insulin resistance in many of these cases of heart failure, independent from its contribution to ischemic heart disease.

The purpose of this review article is to summarize the current evidence for this link between insulin resistance and heart failure. The article is divided into three sections: the first a summary of the epidemiologic and clinical evidence for links between the two diseases, the second a review of the pathophysiologic links between these two diseases, and the third an outline of possible treatment strategies for the insulin resistance seen in heart failure.

Epidemiologic and clinical evidence

In 1974, Kannel and colleagues [1] studied the link between heart failure and diabetes, and found that men who had ischemic cardiomyopathy were more than two times as likely as matched controls to have diabetes mellitus, and women were more than five times as likely. It was, surprisingly, also discovered that the link between diabetes and heart failure actually grew stronger when patients who had ischemic heart disease were excluded [1,2]. Although it is likely with today's modern techniques for investigating the presence or absence of coronary artery disease that some of the nonischemic group of patients would be diagnosed as having ischemic cardiomyopathies, this possibility does not explain why the link would actually become stronger after the removal from the data of patients who had obvious ischemic heart disease. Indeed, in other studies examining the prevalence of diabetes mellitus in idiopathic dilated cardiomyopathy (IDCM), the relative prevalence is much higher, up to 60% to100% more than in a control population [3–9]. In newly diagnosed patients who have heart failure, this prevalence may be up to four times as high [3].

Other major components of the metabolic syndrome, notably hypertension and obesity, are strongly associated with the subsequent development of heart failure and are themselves closely linked to insulin resistance [10–18]. The development of left ventricular (LV) hypertrophy, a strong predictor for the subsequent development of heart failure, is closely linked to insulin resistance also [15,19,20]. The Strong Heart Study in Pima Indians demonstrated that abnormalities of LV size and systolic function correlate with fasting insulin and predate the development of diabetes [21].

* Corresponding author. Division of Cardiovascular Medicine, Stanford University School of Medicine, 300 Pasteur Drive, Falk CVRC 295, Stanford, CA 94305-5406.
E-mail address: mfowler@stanford.edu (M.B. Fowler).

1551-7136/06/$ – see front matter © 2006 Elsevier Inc. All rights reserved.
doi:10.1016/j.hfc.2005.11.007

heartfailure.theclinics.com

Insulin resistance itself has been demonstrated in an IDCM population and can be improved with a regimented exercise program [22]. There is a significant correlation between ejection fraction and insulin resistance, whether or not patients have type 1 diabetes, type 2 diabetes, or normoglycemia [23]. Other evidence points to an 8% increased risk for heart failure for each 1% increase in hemoglobin A1c, even after adjusting for other factors, including ischemic heart disease [24]. Heart failure in diabetic patients carries a particularly poor prognosis, increasing mortality approximately nine-fold [25].

A study by the current authors examined the prevalence of subclinical insulin resistance (rather than overt diabetes) in patients who had IDCM. IDCM patients were significantly insulin-resistant compared with a matched control population, and nearly half of IDCM patients who did not have known diabetes had frank abnormalities of glucose metabolism (Fig. 1) [26]. When patients who had

known diabetes mellitus were included, 59% of IDCM patients had abnormal glucose metabolism. This incidence is even higher than in a recent study of patients who have heart failure in general (ischemic and nonischemic), which found a 43% prevalence of abnormal glucose metabolism [9].

Providing further evidence that insulin resistance is not simply related to coronary ischemia, Swan and colleagues [27] demonstrated that patients who have IDCM are not only more insulin-resistant than healthy controls, but also are more insulin-resistant than patients who have coronary artery disease.

Insulin resistance is correlated with worsened outcomes in nonischemic heart failure. This link is independent of other variables, including the severity of heart failure and maximum oxygen consumption per unit of time (VO_{2max}), suggesting that insulin resistance is more than simply a marker of heart failure itself [28]. Other studies confirmed this finding, noting worsened functional status in patients who have glucose abnormalities, independent of LV ejection fraction [9].

Perhaps one of the strongest pieces of evidence demonstrating a link between insulin resistance and IDCM is that insulin resistance precedes heart failure. In one study, stored blood samples from 20 years before patients developed systolic dysfunction yielded significantly higher proinsulin levels (a surrogate marker for insulin resistance) than in either a healthy population or matched controls [29]. Another study of 1187 Swedish patients who did not have prior heart failure revealed that insulin resistance, independent of all established risk factors (including diabetes mellitus itself), was a major predictor of future heart failure development [10].

The presence or absence of insulin resistance may also predict response to treatment. This situation is not surprising, and in fact would be expected if insulin resistance is part of the pathophysiology of the disease. Carvedilol, which is a potent antiadrenergic agent with insulin-sensitizing properties, has consistently been shown to be effective in preventing mortality in all patients who have heart failure. Patients who have IDCM, however, are up to three times more likely to have a dramatic improvement in LV function in response to carvedilol therapy as those who have ischemic cardiomyopathy [30]. In addition, specific beta-adrenergic genotypes are associated with better or worse responses to antiadrenergic therapy in IDCM [31]. Even more intriguing are recent study results showing that the degree of response to antiadrenergic therapy in IDCM can be predicted by the degree of baseline abnormalities in myocardial glucose uptake [32].

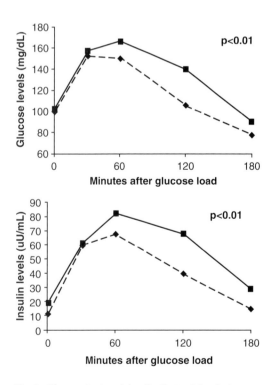

Fig. 1. Glucose (*top*) and insulin (*bottom*) levels in nondiabetic, nonischemic heart failure subjects (*solid line*) versus matched control subjects (dashed line) during an oral glucose tolerance test.

Pathophysiologic links

Energy metabolism

The heart is exquisitely sensitive to its energy requirements, significantly more so than other organs in the body. This sensitivity is caused by the combination of a continuous need for high-energy phosphates to provide energy for contractile function with a limited ability to store substrates. In fact, the heart generates 5 kg/day of ATP, and completely turns over its ATP supply every 13 seconds [33,34].

The heart possesses the ability to oxidize three potential fuels: free fatty acids (FFA), glucose, and lactate [33,35,36]. Of these fuels, FFAs are the predominant substrate for the normal heart, because of the high yield of ATP per molecule of FFA metabolized. Glucose, however, is the more efficient fuel for the heart, because there is a higher yield of ATP per oxygen atom involved in metabolism [37]. Likely for this reason, the heart switches its metabolism toward glucose and away from FFAs in the setting of heart failure, predominantly by downregulating transcription factors for FFA metabolism [33,38–41].

Underlying the use of energy sources is the action of insulin. Insulin binds to insulin receptors, causing autophosphoyrlation of the receptors' regulatory subunits. The activated receptor then phosphorylates a docking protein (insulin receptor substrate-1), which recruits phosphatidylinositol-3 (PI-3) kinase to the plasma membrane [33]. At this point, PI-3 kinase activates the central mediator of insulin's cellular effects, Akt-1 (also known as protein kinase B). Akt-1 activation has numerous consequences, both related to and unrelated to energy metabolism.

Akt-1 activation stimulates nitric oxide production, inhibits apoptosis, and stimulates myocyte hypertrophy [33,42,43]. Therefore, looked at in reverse, lack of insulin responsiveness leads to alterations in myocardial structure, promotion of myocyte apoptosis, and less nitric oxide production (with potential endothelial dysfunction).

The effects of Akt-1 activation on glucose handling are profound, promoting intracellular glucose transport, metabolism, and storage as glycogen [33,42,43]. Insulin's effects on FFA metabolism are the opposite—inhibiting FFA oxidation, and ultimately promoting intramyocardial storage of triacylglycerol. This form of FFA storage is associated with lipotoxicity and worsened heart failure [39,44–47]. In addition, FFAs have been demonstrated to impair Akt-1 activation, promote Akt-1 deactivation, and disrupt intracellular insulin signaling [33,48].

As the heart fails, metabolic pathways become dysregulated, leading to the loss of the heart's ability to switch to its most efficient fuel. Specifically, glucose transporter (GLUT)-1 and peroxisome proliferator activated receptor-α (PPAR-α), vital to glucose and FFA metabolism, respectively, are downregulated, leading to a relative inability to metabolize either fuel [34,40].

Many investigators have noted that the failing heart in many senses recapitulates a fetal gene expression pattern in energy metabolism. In the fetal stages of the developing heart (an oxygen-starved environment, much as in heart failure), glucose is the main energy substrate used, with comparatively little use of FFA [38,49,50]. After birth, a decrease in plasma insulin levels and changes in plasma substrate concentrations lead to relative changes in enzyme production for glucose and FFA metabolism, favoring the use of FFAs. As the heart fails, several changes occur that promote decreased FFA use, increased glucose use, and changes toward fetal isoforms of contractile and calcium regulatory proteins [38, 51,52]. Though the use of energy substrates resembles a fetal pattern, it does so not by upregulation of fetal isoforms, but by downregulation of adult isoforms [53].

The failing heart has significant downregulation of GLUT-1 and GLUT-4, the former being downregulated to a greater extent. There is also concomitant downregulation of pyruvate dehydrogenase kinase (PDK), an enzyme that normally serves to decrease glucose oxidation [40], which explains why the failing heart shifts to greater glucose oxidation despite the downregulation of GLUT-1 and GLUT-4. On the other hand, two main enzymes involved in FFA oxidation—carnitine palmitoyltransferase (CPT)-1 and medium chain acyl-CoA dehydrogenase—are significantly downregulated in the failing human heart, consistent with a switch away from FFA metabolism (Fig. 2) [53,54].

A series of elegant experiments has further defined the importance of energy metabolism in the failing heart. In animal experiments, myocardial underexpression of PPAR-α (causing increased glucose metabolism and decreased FFA metabolism) prevents the development of a diabetic cardiomyopathy, whereas overexpression causes a much more severe cardiomyopathy [47,55]. This cardiomyopathy is reversible by modulating dietary fat content [47]. Treatment with PPAR-γ agonists (agents that promote insulin sensitivity and therefore promote increased glucose and decreased FFA metabolism) prevents the development of systolic dysfunction [47,56–61]. When glucose transporters are overexpressed, ani-

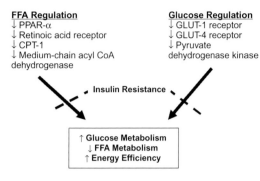

FFA Regulation
↓ PPAR-α
↓ Retinoic acid receptor
↓ CPT-1
↓ Medium-chain acyl CoA
dehydrogenase

Glucose Regulation
↓ GLUT-1 receptor
↓ GLUT-4 receptor
↓ Pyruvate
dehydrogenase kinase

Insulin Resistance

↑ Glucose Metabolism
↓ FFA Metabolism
↑ Energy Efficiency

Fig. 2. Adaptive changes in energy metabolism that are impaired by insulin resistance in the failing heart.

mals are protected from ischemic and nonischemic insults; when they are underexpressed, animals develop much more severe cardiomyopathies [62–65]. In experimentally induced nonischemic heart failure, insulin resistance is seen early and progressively worsens, manifested by high plasma levels of glucose, insulin, FFAs, and norepinephrine [66]. Animals that have cardiomyocyte-selective insulin receptor knockouts have profound changes in energy metabolism, which do not cause significant heart failure in isolation, but leave the heart extremely vulnerable to the addition of any additional stressor, such as increased afterload (Table 1) [67,68].

Leptin-deficient insulin-resistant mice preferentially metabolize FFAs rather than glucose, a situation that is moderately resistant to insulin infusion. Moreover, the hearts in these insulin-resistant mice are less efficient, with myocardial oxygen consumption ranging from 30% to 100% higher than wild-type mice [69]. Rats that have insulin resistance (but not diabetes) from high-sucrose feeding develop myocardial dysfunction, which is preventable and reversible with multiple lines of therapy aimed at treating insulin resistance (exercise, metformin, troglitazone), but not by therapy (sulfonylureas) that treats hyperglycemia without treating insulin resistance [70–73].

It is probable that in the failing heart, which attempts to switch to an energy-using program of greater glucose oxidation and less FFA oxidation, the actions of insulin (which promote this switch) are critically important. Specifically, at a critical pathophysiologic moment when the heart needs to maximize energy efficiency, insulin resistance can interfere with its doing so. It is in this context, therefore, that a link between myocardial resistance and insulin's actions could contribute to the development and worsening of heart failure.

Energy deficit and uncoupling proteins

Another intriguing hypothesis linking insulin resistance and heart failure involves mitochondrial uncoupling proteins present in the myocardium. The failing heart is in a state of energy deficit, demonstrable by low myocardial phosphocreatine to ATP

Table 1
Models for interactions among insulin resistance, energy metabolism, and heart failure

Model/therapy	Metabolic change	Result
Underexpression PPAR-α	↓ FFA metabolism ↑ Glucose metabolism	Protection from diabetic CM
Overexpression PPAR-α	↑ FFA metabolism ↓ Glucose metabolism	Promotes diabetic CM
Overexpression PPAR-α and high-fat diet	↑ Myocardial triglyceride accumulation	Promotes diabetic CM and reversible with diet change
PPAR-γ agonist therapy	↑ Insulin sensitivity ↑ Glucose metabolism	Prevents LV dysfunction in ischemic and nonischemic CM
Myocardial PPAR-γ knockout	↓ Akt phosphorylation	Diastolic dysfunction and myocyte hypertrophy
Carvedilol therapy	↓ FFA metabolism ↑ Myocardial efficiency	Improved LV function, especially in nonischemic CM
GLUT-1 overexpression	↑ Glucose metabolism ↑ Energy reserve	Protection from pressure-induced LV dysfunction
GLUT-4 knockout	↓ Glucose metabolism	Promotes LV dysfunction with hypoxic insult
Leptin deficiency	↑ FFA metabolism ↓ Glucose metabolism	↓ Energy efficiency and ↑ oxygen consumption
Myocardial insulin receptor knockout	↓ Insulin sensitivity ↓ FFA metabolism ↑ Glucose metabolism	Baseline LV dysfunction, profound LV dysfunction with increased afterload

Abbreviations: CM, cardiomyopathy; ↑, increased; ↓, decreased.

ratios; this deficit corresponds to increased mortality [74]. Much of this energy deficit is because of profound energy wasting, caused by increased transcription of uncoupling proteins (which cause the mitochondria to produce heat rather than ATP). Intriguingly, the elevated FFA levels and the low GLUT-4 levels seen in insulin resistance are associated with increased transcription of uncoupling proteins [75,76].

Sympathetic nervous system activation and the diabetic heart

Diabetes is associated with classic histopathologic changes in the heart, most notably with myocyte loss, replacement fibrosis, and accumulation of periodic acid-Schiff–positive material [77–79]. Increased rates of apoptosis have also been observed in the myocardium of diabetic hearts [80]. Many of these changes are also seen in states of catecholamine excess (eg, pheochromocytomas, beta-receptor over-expressing animals) [81]. Notably, insulin resistance and heart failure are both associated with catecholamine excess.

Activation of the sympathetic nervous system serves to further the cellular effects of insulin resistance, in addition to increasing myocardial energy demand. Catecholamines directly antagonize insulin's actions and promote lipolysis, which increases circulating FFAs with a resultant furthering of insulin resistance [82,83]. Insulin therapy has been shown to reduce the extent of catecholamine-induced myocardial damage in the heart [84]. The potent sympathetic nervous system blocker carvedilol reduces myocardial FFA use, with a resultant improvement in myocardial efficiency [85].

A recent study has shed further light on the role of the sympathetic nervous system in promoting myocardial insulin resistance. Though short-term beta-receptor stimulation promotes insulin-mediated myocardial glucose uptake, long-term beta-receptor stimulation inhibits both insulin-mediated myocardial glucose uptake and activation of the insulin receptor [86]. This mechanism provides a plausible means by which beta-adrenergic blocking medications may exert a particularly profound effect in patients who have cardiomyopathies caused by insulin resistance.

Diastolic dysfunction: the first manifestation of insulin resistance?

Animals and humans who have diabetes, or even subclinical insulin resistance, have abnormal diastolic heart function [87–94]. The presence of insulin resistance itself promotes diastolic dysfunction independent of other variables, including hypertension [95]. It is likely that this diastolic dysfunction is a common early manifestation of insulin resistance in the heart, and one that is far more common than systolic heart failure, which strikes a much smaller percentage of individuals. Many patients who have supposedly normal systolic function have abnormalities demonstrated when the heart is under stress [94,96–98]. Mice that have myocardial PPAR-γ knockouts (a model for myocardial insulin resistance) develop myocardial hypertrophy, even without an additional insult, and have demonstrable diastolic dysfunction on echocardiography [99]. Underscoring the importance of insulin's actions in diabetic hearts, insulin has been found to be a potent inotrope in diabetic hearts, whereas it has no effect on normal hearts [100,101].

Inflammation

Another potential link between insulin resistance and heart failure is through dysregulation of inflammatory mediators. Heart failure is a hyperinflammatory state. Multiple mediators of inflammation are upregulated in heart failure, including in patients who have IDCM [102–106]. An excess of inflammatory mediators can cause a nonischemic cardiomyopathy, whereas antagonism can prevent a cardiomyopathy [107–110]. Though large-scale clinical trials of inflammatory-modulating agents have been unsuccessful at changing heart failure outcomes, it is possible that this result is because the trials have targeted individual components of the inflammatory cascade (eg, endothelin, tumor necrosis factor-α) rather than an underlying mediator of inflammatory pathways, such as insulin resistance [111,112]. Insulin resistance produces an inflammatory state by upregulating the same inflammatory mediators seen in heart failure, and this state can be counteracted by treatment with insulin-sensitizing medications [113,114].

Potential therapy targets to treat insulin resistance

Many of the therapies that are considered standard in the treatment of heart failure have significant effects on glucose metabolism and insulin sensitivity. Standard lifestyle recommendations (weight loss, aerobic exercise, smoking cessation) are all associated with improved insulin sensitivity [115–117]. Indeed, exercise itself improves insulin resistance and outcomes in heart failure [22].

Beta-blocking medications are now considered standard therapy for heart failure, though with considerable variation among the specific medications in this class. Metoprolol, bisoprolol, and carvedilol have all shown mortality benefits in heart failure, whereas bucindolol has not [118–123]. One important area of difference among different beta-blocking medications is their effects on insulin sensitivity, with carvedilol having either a neutral or insulin-sensitizing effect, and the others (including metoprolol) having significant effects promoting insulin resistance [123–128]. Though head-to-head comparisons between carvedilol and metoprolol have found better metabolic effects and better outcomes with carvedilol, it is unknown if the metabolic/insulin-sensitizing effects are the reason for the difference.

Other therapies that have proven mortality benefits in heart failure and are now considered standard therapy almost all appear to have beneficial metabolic effects. In particular, angiotensin-converting enzyme inhibitors, angiotensin receptor blockers, aldosterone antagonists, and statins all have beneficial effects on glucose metabolism and insulin sensitivity [129–133]. On the other hand, diuretics, particularly thiazide diuretics, cause worsened insulin resistance and glucose metabolism [134].

Conceptually, it should be possible to affect outcomes by treating patients who have insulin resistance and cardiomyopathy with an insulin-sensitizing medication. Of these, the two most promising medications are metformin and the thiazolidinediones. Metformin has been demonstrated to prevent worsened glucose metabolism in an insulin resistant non-heart-failure population [117]. In addition, metformin has beneficial effects on calcium handling in cardiac myocytes [72]. In a positron emission tomography study examining myocardial glucose uptake, however, the thiazolidinedione medication rosiglitazone improved myocardial glucose uptake (likely a result of FFA suppression), whereas metformin had no effect [58]. Given the important observations noted above that the thiazolidinediones (PPARγ agonists) can prevent and reverse "diabetic cardiomyopathy" in animals, this area is clearly ripe for further exploration [60,61].

Though thiazolidinediones can be associated with increased peripheral edema, current consensus guidelines support their use in compensated heart failure [135]. Preliminary results of a small trial studying the use of rosiglitazone in patients who had diabetes and either ischemic or nonischemic heart failure were presented at the 2005 American Diabetes Association annual meeting. The study demonstrated adequate safety of rosiglitazone in this population, but no significant change in ejection fraction was seen. An ongoing National Institutes of Health (NIH) Phase II clinical study is examining the role of rosiglitazone in the treatment of heart failure in patients who have either type 2 diabetes or glucose intolerance [136]. Future studies that specifically target a patient population whose heart failure is caused by a cardiomyopathy as a result of insulin resistance may be needed to demonstrate an important therapeutic benefit.

Summary

1. Epidemiologic and clinical evidence reveals that insulin resistance is strikingly abundant in the heart failure population, predates the heart failure itself, independently portends a worse prognosis, and predicts a greater clinical response to antiadrenergic therapy.

2. The heart's response to many forms of injury or insult is one of increased glucose use, decreased FFA use, and increased energy efficiency. The heart's response to insulin resistance is one of decreased glucose use, increased FFA use, and decreased energy efficiency—precisely the opposite adaptations as that of the injury/insult response. The combined states of insulin resistance and heart failure produce a "starved myocardium," in a sense allowing the heart to drown in a sea of available substrates that it is unable to use.

3. Myocardial insulin resistance has other negative effects on the myocardium, including blunted nitric oxide production, promotion of apoptosis, and increased catecholamine-mediated damage.

4. Almost all current heart failure therapies also concurrently improve insulin sensitivity. Whether therapy specifically directed at improving insulin sensitivity will improve heart failure outcomes is currently unknown.

5. The current authors postulate that in some patients who have IDCM and in whom other causes of nonischemic dilated cardiomyopathy can be excluded, insulin resistance has a primary causative role in the development of their cardiomyopathy and heart failure. These patients with an "Insulin-Resistant Cardiomyopathy" characteristically normalize LV ejection fraction after therapy with beta-blocking medications, continue to exhibit features of impaired myocardial relaxation, and frequently develop overt diabetes in the future (RMW and MBF, unpublished observations, 2005).

Recognition of the effects of insulin resistance on the pathogenesis and progression of heart failure has long suffered from an embarrassment of riches. Links between insulin resistance and ischemic heart disease, and between ischemic heart disease and heart failure, are undeniably present and have been the focus of most of the investigations into these two diseases. It is now clear, however, that an even more fundamental link exists. The failing heart needs to use energy more efficiently than the nonfailing heart; adaptive changes in metabolism attempt to do just that. It is the exact time when insulin resistance— which at its most fundamental level interferes with efficient energy metabolism—can wreak havoc on the failing heart. Basic science and clinical evidence now support a link between insulin resistance and the pathogenesis/progression of heart failure, one which provides potential treatment targets for the future. An understanding of these relationships already sheds new light on some of the successes of current heart failure therapy and clearly opens the door for future investigations. As the links between insulin resistance and heart failure become clear, investigations into these two diseases may at last be converging.

References

[1] Kannel WB, Hjortland M, Castelli WP. Role of diabetes in congestive heart failure: the Framingham study. Am J Cardiol 1974;34(1):29–34.

[2] Zarich SW, Nesto RW. Diabetic cardiomyopathy. Am Heart J 1989;118(5 Pt 1):1000–12.

[3] Amato L, Paolisso G, Cacciatore F, et al. Congestive heart failure predicts the development of non-insulin-dependent diabetes mellitus in the elderly. The Osservatorio Geriatrico Regione Campania Group. Diabetes Metab 1997;23(3):213–8.

[4] Bertoni AG, Tsai A, Kasper EK, et al. Diabetes and idiopathic cardiomyopathy: a nationwide case-control study. Diabetes Care 2003;26(10):2791–5.

[5] Hamby RI, Zoneraich S, Sherman L. Diabetic cardiomyopathy. JAMA 1974;229(13):1749–54.

[6] Shapiro LM, Howat AP, Calter MM. Left ventricular function in diabetes mellitus. I: Methodology, and prevalence and spectrum of abnormalities. Br Heart J 1981;45(2):122–8.

[7] Shapiro LM, Leatherdale BA, Coyne ME, et al. Prospective study of heart disease in untreated maturity onset diabetics. Br Heart J 1980;44(3):342–8.

[8] Shapiro LM, Leatherdale BA, Mackinnon J, et al. Left ventricular function in diabetes mellitus. II: Relation between clinical features and left ventricular function. Br Heart J 1981;45(2):129–32.

[9] Suskin N, McKelvie RS, Burns RJ, et al. Glucose and insulin abnormalities relate to functional ca-

[10] Ingelsson E, Sundstrom J, Arnlov J, et al. Insulin resistance and risk of congestive heart failure. JAMA 2005;294(3):334–41.

[11] Ho KK, Pinsky JL, Kannel WB, et al. The epidemiology of heart failure: the Framingham Study. J Am Coll Cardiol 1993;22(4)(Suppl A):6A–13A.

[12] Chen YT, Vaccarino V, Williams CS, et al. Risk factors for heart failure in the elderly: a prospective community-based study. Am J Med 1999;106(6):605–12.

[13] Gottdiener JS, Arnold AM, Aurigemma GP, et al. Predictors of congestive heart failure in the elderly: the Cardiovascular Health Study. J Am Coll Cardiol 2000;35(6):1628–37.

[14] He J, Ogden LG, Bazzano LA, et al. Risk factors for congestive heart failure in US men and women: NHANES I epidemiologic follow-up study. Arch Intern Med 2001;161(7):996–1002.

[15] Kannel WB, Castelli WP, McNamara PM, et al. Role of blood pressure in the development of congestive heart failure. The Framingham study. N Engl J Med 1972;287(16):781–7.

[16] Levy D, Larson MG, Vasan RS, et al. The progression from hypertension to congestive heart failure. JAMA 1996;275(20):1557–62.

[17] Kenchaiah S, Evans JC, Levy D, et al. Obesity and the risk of heart failure. N Engl J Med 2002;347(5):305–13.

[18] Wilhelmsen L, Rosengren A, Eriksson H, et al. Heart failure in the general population of men—morbidity, risk factors and prognosis. J Intern Med 2001;249(3):253–61.

[19] Kannel WB, Levy D, Cupples LA. Left ventricular hypertrophy and risk of cardiac failure: insights from the Framingham Study. J Cardiovasc Pharmacol 1987;10(Suppl 6):S135.

[20] Verdecchia P, Reboldi G, Schillaci G, et al. Circulating insulin and insulin growth factor-1 are independent determinants of left ventricular mass and geometry in essential hypertension. Circulation 1999;100(17):1802–7.

[21] Ilercil A, Devereux RB, Roman MJ, et al. Associations of insulin levels with left ventricular structure and function in American Indians: the Strong Heart Study. Diabetes 2002;51(5):1543–7.

[22] Kemppainen J, Tsuchida H, Stolen K, et al. Insulin signalling and resistance in patients with chronic heart failure. J Physiol 2003;550(Pt 1):305–15.

[23] Iozzo P, Chareonthaitawee P, Dutka D, et al. Independent association of type 2 diabetes and coronary artery disease with myocardial insulin resistance. Diabetes 2002;51(10):3020–4.

[24] Iribarren C, Karter AJ, Go AS, et al. Glycemic control and heart failure among adult patients with diabetes. Circulation 2001;103(22):2668–73.

[25] Bertoni AG, Hundley WG, Massing MW, et al. Heart failure prevalence, incidence, and mortality in the

elderly with diabetes. Diabetes Care 2004;27(3): 699–703.

[26] Witteles RM, Tang WH, Jamali AH, et al. Insulin resistance in idiopathic dilated cardiomyopathy: a possible etiologic link. J Am Coll Cardiol 2004; 44(1):78–81.

[27] Swan JW, Anker SD, Walton C, et al. Insulin resistance in chronic heart failure: relation to severity and etiology of heart failure. J Am Coll Cardiol 1997;30(2):527–32.

[28] Paolisso G, Tagliamonte MR, Rizzo MR, et al. Prognostic importance of insulin-mediated glucose uptake in aged patients with congestive heart failure secondary to mitral and/or aortic valve disease. Am J Cardiol 1999;83(9):1338–44.

[29] Arnlov J, Lind L, Zethelius B, et al. Several factors associated with the insulin resistance syndrome are predictors of left ventricular systolic dysfunction in a male population after 20 years of follow-up. Am Heart J 2001;142(4):720–4.

[30] O'Keefe Jr JH, Magalski A, Stevens TL, et al. Predictors of improvement in left ventricular ejection fraction with carvedilol for congestive heart failure. J Nucl Cardiol 2000;7(1):3–7.

[31] Kaye DM, Smirk B, Williams C, et al. Beta-adrenoceptor genotype influences the response to carvedilol in patients with congestive heart failure. Pharmacogenetics 2003;13(7):379–82.

[32] Hasegawa S, Kusuoka H, Maruyama K, et al. Myocardial positron emission computed tomographic images obtained with fluorine-18 fluoro-2-deoxyglucose predict the response of idiopathic dilated cardiomyopathy patients to beta-blockers. J Am Coll Cardiol 2004;43(2):224–33.

[33] Shah A, Shannon RP. Insulin resistance in dilated cardiomyopathy. Rev Cardiovasc Med 2003;4(Suppl 6): S50–7.

[34] Taegtmeyer H. Switching metabolic genes to build a better heart. Circulation 2002;106(16):2043–5.

[35] Taegtmeyer H, McNulty P, Young ME. Adaptation and maladaptation of the heart in diabetes: part I: general concepts. Circulation 2002;105(14): 1727–33.

[36] Young ME, McNulty P, Taegtmeyer H. Adaptation and maladaptation of the heart in diabetes: part II: potential mechanisms. Circulation 2002;105(15): 1861–70.

[37] Opie L. The heart: physiology and metabolism. New York: Raven Press; 1991.

[38] Davila-Roman VG, Vedala G, Herrero P, et al. Altered myocardial fatty acid and glucose metabolism in idiopathic dilated cardiomyopathy. J Am Coll Cardiol 2002;40(2):271–7.

[39] Osorio JC, Stanley WC, Linke A, et al. Impaired myocardial fatty acid oxidation and reduced protein expression of retinoid X receptor-alpha in pacing-induced heart failure. Circulation 2002;106(5):606–12.

[40] Razeghi P, Young ME, Cockrill TC, et al. Down-regulation of myocardial myocyte enhancer factor 2C and myocyte enhancer factor 2C-regulated gene expression in diabetic patients with nonischemic heart failure. Circulation 2002;106(4):407–11.

[41] Taegtmeyer H, Hems R, Krebs HA. Utilization of energy-providing substrates in the isolated working rat heart. Biochem J 1980;186(3):701–11.

[42] Brazil DP, Hemmings BA. Ten years of protein kinase B signalling: a hard Akt to follow. Trends Biochem Sci 2001;26(11):657–64.

[43] Lawlor MA, Alessi DR. PKB/Akt: a key mediator of cell proliferation, survival and insulin responses? J Cell Sci 2001;114(Pt 16):2903–10.

[44] Bonnet D, Martin D, Pascale De L, et al. Arrhythmias and conduction defects as presenting symptoms of fatty acid oxidation disorders in children. Circulation 1999;100(22):2248–53.

[45] Chiu HC, Kovacs A, Ford DA, et al. A novel mouse model of lipotoxic cardiomyopathy. J Clin Invest 2001;107(7):813–22.

[46] Corr PB, Creer MH, Yamada KA, et al. Prophylaxis of early ventricular fibrillation by inhibition of acyl-carnitine accumulation. J Clin Invest 1989;83(3): 927–36.

[47] Finck BN, Han X, Courtois M, et al. A critical role for PPARalpha-mediated lipotoxicity in the pathogenesis of diabetic cardiomyopathy: modulation by dietary fat content. Proc Natl Acad Sci U S A 2003; 100(3):1226–31.

[48] Birnbaum MJ. Turning down insulin signaling. J Clin Invest 2001;108(5):655–9.

[49] Kantor PF, Robertson MA, Coe JY, et al. Volume overload hypertrophy of the newborn heart slows the maturation of enzymes involved in the regulation of fatty acid metabolism. J Am Coll Cardiol 1999; 33(6):1724–34.

[50] Lopaschuk GD, Collins-Nakai RL, Itoi T. Developmental changes in energy substrate use by the heart. Cardiovasc Res 1992;26(12):1172–80.

[51] Barger PM, Kelly DP. Fatty acid utilization in the hypertrophied and failing heart: molecular regulatory mechanisms. Am J Med Sci 1999;318(1):36–42.

[52] Sack MN, Rader TA, Park S, et al. Fatty acid oxidation enzyme gene expression is downregulated in the failing heart. Circulation 1996;94(11): 2837–42.

[53] Razeghi P, Young ME, Alcorn JL, et al. Metabolic gene expression in fetal and failing human heart. Circulation 2001;104(24):2923–31.

[54] Martin MA, Gomez MA, Guillen F, et al. Myocardial carnitine and carnitine palmitoyltransferase deficiencies in patients with severe heart failure. Biochimica et Biophysica Acta 2000;1502(3):330–6.

[55] Finck BN, Lehman JJ, Leone TC, et al. The cardiac phenotype induced by PPARalpha overexpression mimics that caused by diabetes mellitus. J Clin Invest 2002;109(1):121–30.

[56] Shiomi T, Tsutsui H, Hayashidani S, et al. Pioglitazone, a peroxisome proliferator-activated receptor-gamma agonist, attenuates left ventricular remodeling

and failure after experimental myocardial infarction. Circulation 2002;106(24):3126–32.

[57] Carley AN, Semeniuk LM, Shimoni Y, et al. Treatment of type 2 diabetic db/db mice with a novel PPARgamma agonist improves cardiac metabolism but not contractile function. Am J Physiol Endocrinol Metab 2004;286(3):E449–55.

[58] Hallsten K, Virtanen KA, Lonnqvist F, et al. Enhancement of insulin-stimulated myocardial glucose uptake in patients with Type 2 diabetes treated with rosiglitazone. Diabet Med 2004;21(12):1280–7.

[59] Liu LS, Tanaka H, Ishii S, et al. The new antidiabetic drug MCC-555 acutely sensitizes insulin signaling in isolated cardiomyocytes. Endocrinology 1998;139(11):4531–9.

[60] Sidell RJ, Cole MA, Draper NJ, et al. Thiazolidinedione treatment normalizes insulin resistance and ischemic injury in the Zucker fatty rat heart. Diabetes 2002;51(4):1110–7.

[61] Zhou YT, Grayburn P, Karim A, et al. Lipotoxic heart disease in obese rats: implications for human obesity. Proc Natl Acad Sci U S A 2000;97(4):1784–9.

[62] Abel ED, Kaulbach HC, Tian R, et al. Cardiac hypertrophy with preserved contractile function after selective deletion of GLUT4 from the heart. J Clin Invest 1999;104(12):1703–14.

[63] Liao R, Jain M, Cui L, et al. Cardiac-specific overexpression of GLUT1 prevents the development of heart failure attributable to pressure overload in mice. Circulation 2002;106(16):2125–31.

[64] Minokoshi Y, Kahn CR, Kahn BB. Tissue-specific ablation of the GLUT4 glucose transporter or the insulin receptor challenges assumptions about insulin action and glucose homeostasis. J Biol Chem 2003;278(36):33609–12.

[65] Tian R, Abel ED. Responses of GLUT4-deficient hearts to ischemia underscore the importance of glycolysis. Circulation 2001;103(24):2961–6.

[66] Nikolaidis LA, Sturzu A, Stolarski C, et al. The development of myocardial insulin resistance in conscious dogs with advanced dilated cardiomyopathy. Cardiovasc Res 2004;61(2):297–306.

[67] Belke DD, Betuing S, Tuttle MJ, et al. Insulin signaling coordinately regulates cardiac size, metabolism, and contractile protein isoform expression. J Clin Invest 2002;109(5):629–39.

[68] Hu P, Zhang D, Swenson L, et al. Minimally invasive aortic banding in mice: effects of altered cardiomyocyte insulin signaling during pressure overload. Am J Physiol Heart Circ Physiol 2003;285(3):H1261–9.

[69] Mazumder PK, O'Neill BT, Roberts MW, et al. Impaired cardiac efficiency and increased fatty acid oxidation in insulin-resistant ob/ob mouse hearts. Diabetes 2004;53(9):2366–74.

[70] Dutta K, Podolin DA, Davidson MB, et al. Cardiomyocyte dysfunction in sucrose-fed rats is associated with insulin resistance. Diabetes 2001;50(5):1186–92.

[71] Davidoff AJ, Mason MM, Davidson MB, et al. Sucrose-induced cardiomyocyte dysfunction is both preventable and reversible with clinically relevant treatments. Am J Physiol Endocrinol Metab 2004;286(5):E718–24.

[72] Ren J, Dominguez LJ, Sowers JR, et al. Metformin but not glyburide prevents high glucose-induced abnormalities in relaxation and intracellular Ca2 + transients in adult rat ventricular myocytes. Diabetes 1999;48(10):2059–65.

[73] Ren J, Dominguez LJ, Sowers JR, et al. Troglitazone attenuates high-glucose-induced abnormalities in relaxation and intracellular calcium in rat ventricular myocytes. Diabetes 1996;45(12):1822–5.

[74] Neubauer S, Horn M, Cramer M, et al. Myocardial phosphocreatine-to-ATP ratio is a predictor of mortality in patients with dilated cardiomyopathy. Circulation 1997;96(7):2190–6.

[75] Murray AJ, Anderson RE, Watson GC, et al. Uncoupling proteins in human heart. Lancet 2004;364(9447):1786–8.

[76] Opie LH. The metabolic vicious cycle in heart failure. Lancet 2004;364(9447):1733–4.

[77] Nunoda S, Genda A, Sugihara N, et al. Quantitative approach to the histopathology of the biopsied right ventricular myocardium in patients with diabetes mellitus. Heart Vessels 1985;1(1):43–7.

[78] Regan TJ, Lyons MM, Ahmed SS, et al. Evidence for cardiomyopathy in familial diabetes mellitus. J Clin Invest 1977;60(4):884–99.

[79] Vitolo E, Madoi S, Sponzilli C, et al. Vectorcardiographic evaluation of diabetic cardiomyopathy and of its contributing factors. Acta Diabetologica Latina 1988;25(3):227–34.

[80] Frustaci A, Kajstura J, Chimenti C, et al. Myocardial cell death in human diabetes. Circ Res 2000;87(12):1123–32.

[81] Liggett SB, Tepe NM, Lorenz JN, et al. Early and delayed consequences of beta(2)-adrenergic receptor overexpression in mouse hearts: critical role for expression level. Circulation 2000;101(14):1707–14.

[82] Nonogaki K. New insights into sympathetic regulation of glucose and fat metabolism. Diabetologia 2000;43(5):533–49.

[83] Hjemdahl P. Stress and the metabolic syndrome: an interesting but enigmatic association. Circulation 2002;106(21):2634–6.

[84] Downing SE, Lee JC. Effects of insulin on experimental catecholamine cardiomyopathy. Am J Pathol 1978;93(2):339–52.

[85] Wallhaus TR, Taylor M, DeGrado TR, et al. Myocardial free fatty acid and glucose use after carvedilol treatment in patients with congestive heart failure. Circulation 2001;103(20):2441–6.

[86] Morisco C, Condorelli G, Trimarco V, et al. Akt mediates the cross-talk between beta-adrenergic and insulin receptors in neonatal cardiomyocytes. Circ Res 2005;96(2):180–8.

[87] Andersen NH, Poulsen SH, Eiskjaer H, et al. Decreased left ventricular longitudinal contraction

in normotensive and normoalbuminuric patients with type II diabetes mellitus: a doppler tissue tracking and strain rate echocardiography study. Clin Sci (Lond) 2003;105(1):59–66.

[88] Andersen NH, Poulsen SH, Poulsen PL, et al. Left ventricular dysfunction in hypertensive patients with type 2 diabetes mellitus. Diabet Med 2005;22(9):1218–25.

[89] Vinereanu D, Nicolaides E, Tweddel AC, et al. Subclinical left ventricular dysfunction in asymptomatic patients with type II diabetes mellitus, related to serum lipids and glycated haemoglobin. Clin Sci (Lond) 2003;105(5):591–9.

[90] Cosson S, Kevorkian JP. Left ventricular diastolic dysfunction: an early sign of diabetic cardiomyopathy? Diabetes Metab 2003;29(5):455–66.

[91] Schannwell CM, Schneppenheim M, Perings S, et al. Left ventricular diastolic dysfunction as an early manifestation of diabetic cardiomyopathy. Cardiology 2002;98(1–2):33–9.

[92] Poirier P, Bogaty P, Garneau C, et al. Diastolic dysfunction in normotensive men with well-controlled type 2 diabetes: importance of maneuvers in echocardiographic screening for preclinical diabetic cardiomyopathy. Diabetes Care 2001;24(1):5–10.

[93] Zabalgoitia M, Ismaeil MF, Anderson L, et al. Prevalence of diastolic dysfunction in normotensive, asymptomatic patients with well-controlled type 2 diabetes mellitus. Am J Cardiol 2001;87(3):320–3.

[94] Fang ZY, Yuda S, Anderson V, et al. Echocardiographic detection of early diabetic myocardial disease. J Am Coll Cardiol 2003;41(4):611–7.

[95] Mizushige K, Yao L, Noma T, et al. Alteration in left ventricular diastolic filling and accumulation of myocardial collagen at insulin-resistant prediabetic stage of a type II diabetic rat model. Circulation 2000;101(8):899–907.

[96] Carlstrom S, Karlefors T. Haemodynamic studies on newly diagnosed diabetics before and after adequate insulin treatment. Br Heart J 1970;32(3):355–8.

[97] Karlefors T. Haemodynamic studies in male diabetics. Acta Medica Scandinavica Supplementum 1966;449:45–80.

[98] Vered A, Battler A, Segal P, et al. Exercise-induced left ventricular dysfunction in young men with asymptomatic diabetes mellitus (diabetic cardiomyopathy). Am J Cardiol 1984;54(6):633–7.

[99] Duan SZ, Ivashchenko CY, Russell MW, et al. Cardiomyocyte-specific knockout and agonist of peroxisome proliferator-activated receptor-gamma both induce cardiac hypertrophy in mice. Circ Res 2005;97(4):372–9.

[100] Ren J, Walsh MF, Hamaty M, et al. Augmentation of the inotropic response to insulin in diabetic rat hearts. Life Sci 1999;65(4):369–80.

[101] Williams RS, Schaible TF, Scheuer J, et al. Effects of experimental diabetes on adrenergic and cholinergic receptors of rat myocardium. Diabetes 1983;32(10):881–6.

[102] Stewart DJ, Cernacek P, Costello KB, et al. Elevated endothelin-1 in heart failure and loss of normal response to postural change. Circulation 1992;85(2):510–7.

[103] Yanagisawa M, Kurihara H, Kimura S, et al. A novel potent vasoconstrictor peptide produced by vascular endothelial cells. Nature 1988;332(6163):411–5.

[104] Sakai S, Miyauchi T, Sakurai T, et al. Endogenous endothelin-1 participates in the maintenance of cardiac function in rats with congestive heart failure. Marked increase in endothelin-1 production in the failing heart. Circulation 1996;93(6):1214–22.

[105] Picard P, Smith PJ, Monge JC, et al. Coordinated upregulation of the cardiac endothelin system in a rat model of heart failure. J Cardiovasc Pharmacol 1998;31(Suppl 1):S294–7.

[106] Pieske B, Beyermann B, Breu V, et al. Functional effects of endothelin and regulation of endothelin receptors in isolated human nonfailing and failing myocardium. Circulation 1999;99(14):1802–9.

[107] Yang LL, Gros R, Kabir MG, et al. Conditional cardiac overexpression of endothelin-1 induces inflammation and dilated cardiomyopathy in mice. Circulation 2004;109(2):255–61.

[108] Fraccarollo D, Hu K, Galuppo P, et al. Chronic endothelin receptor blockade attenuates progressive ventricular dilation and improves cardiac function in rats with myocardial infarction: possible involvement of myocardial endothelin system in ventricular remodeling. Circulation 1997;96(11):3963–73.

[109] Kubota T, McTiernan CF, Frye CS, et al. Dilated cardiomyopathy in transgenic mice with cardiac-specific overexpression of tumor necrosis factor-alpha. Circ Res 1997;81(4):627–35.

[110] Bozkurt B, Kribbs SB, Clubb Jr FJ, et al. Pathophysiologically relevant concentrations of tumor necrosis factor-alpha promote progressive left ventricular dysfunction and remodeling in rats. Circulation 1998;97(14):1382–91.

[111] Chung ES, Packer M, Lo KH, et al. Randomized, double-blind, placebo-controlled, pilot trial of infliximab, a chimeric monoclonal antibody to tumor necrosis factor-alpha, in patients with moderate-to-severe heart failure: results of the anti-TNF Therapy Against Congestive Heart Failure (ATTACH) trial. Circulation 2003;107(25):3133–40.

[112] Kalra PR, Moon JC, Coats AJ. Do results of the ENABLE (Endothelin Antagonist Bosentan for Lowering Cardiac Events in Heart Failure) study spell the end for non-selective endothelin antagonism in heart failure? Int J Cardiol 2002;85(2–3):195–7.

[113] Itoh H, Doi K, Tanaka T, et al. Hypertension and insulin resistance: role of peroxisome proliferator-activated receptor gamma. Clin Exp Pharmacol Physiol 1999;26(7):558–60.

[114] Winkler G, Lakatos P, Salamon F, et al. Elevated serum TNF-alpha level as a link between endothelial dysfunction and insulin resistance in normotensive obese patients. Diabet Med 1999;16(3):207–11.

[115] Tuomilehto J, Lindstrom J, Eriksson JG, et al. Prevention of type 2 diabetes mellitus by changes in lifestyle among subjects with impaired glucose tolerance. N Engl J Med 2001;344(18):1343–50.

[116] Wannamethee SG, Shaper AG, Perry IJ. Smoking as a modifiable risk factor for type 2 diabetes in middle-aged men. Diabetes Care 2001;24(9):1590–5.

[117] Knowler WC, Barrett-Connor E, Fowler SE, et al. Reduction in the incidence of type 2 diabetes with lifestyle intervention or metformin. N Engl J Med 2002;346(6):393–403.

[118] The Cardiac Insufficiency Bisoprolol Study II (CIBIS-II). A randomised trial. Lancet 1999;353(9146): 9–13.

[119] The Beta-Blocker Evaluation of Survival Trial Investigators. A trial of the beta-blocker bucindolol in patients with advanced chronic heart failure. N Engl J Med 2001;344(22):1659–67.

[120] Effect of metoprolol CR/XL in chronic heart failure: Metoprolol CR/XL Randomised Intervention Trial in Congestive Heart Failure (MERIT-HF). Lancet 1999;353(9169):2001–7.

[121] Packer M, Bristow MR, Cohn JN, et al. The effect of carvedilol on morbidity and mortality in patients with chronic heart failure. US Carvedilol Heart Failure Study Group. N Engl J Med 1996;334(21): 1349–55.

[122] Packer M, Coats AJ, Fowler MB, et al. Effect of carvedilol on survival in severe chronic heart failure. N Engl J Med 2001;344(22):1651–8.

[123] Packer M, Antonopoulos GV, Berlin JA, et al. Comparative effects of carvedilol and metoprolol on left ventricular ejection fraction in heart failure: results of a meta-analysis. Am Heart J 2001;141(6): 899–907.

[124] Bakris GL, Fonseca V, Katholi RE, et al. Metabolic effects of carvedilol vs metoprolol in patients with type 2 diabetes mellitus and hypertension: a randomized controlled trial. JAMA 2004;292(18): 2227–36.

[125] Ferrua S, Bobbio M, Catalano E, et al. Does carvedilol impair insulin sensitivity in heart failure patients without diabetes? J Card Fail 2005;11(8): 590–4.

[126] Jacob S, Rett K, Wicklmayr M, et al. Differential effect of chronic treatment with two beta-blocking agents on insulin sensitivity: the carvedilol-metoprolol study. J Hypertens 1996;14(4):489–94.

[127] Poole-Wilson PA, Swedberg K, Cleland JG, et al. Comparison of carvedilol and metoprolol on clinical outcomes in patients with chronic heart failure in the Carvedilol Or Metoprolol European Trial (COMET): randomised controlled trial. Lancet 2003;362(9377): 7–13.

[128] Sanderson JE, Chan SK, Yip G, et al. Beta-blockade in heart failure: a comparison of carvedilol with metoprolol. J Am Coll Cardiol 1999;34(5):1522–8.

[129] Dahlof B, Devereux RB, Kjeldsen SE, et al. Cardiovascular morbidity and mortality in the Losartan Intervention For Endpoint reduction in hypertension study (LIFE): a randomised trial against atenolol. Lancet 2002;359(9311):995–1003.

[130] Freeman DJ, Norrie J, Sattar N, et al. Pravastatin and the development of diabetes mellitus: evidence for a protective treatment effect in the West of Scotland Coronary Prevention Study. Circulation 2001;103(3): 357–62.

[131] Hansson L, Lindholm LH, Niskanen L, et al. Effect of angiotensin-converting-enzyme inhibition compared with conventional therapy on cardiovascular morbidity and mortality in hypertension: the Captopril Prevention Project (CAPPP) randomised trial. Lancet 1999;353(9153):611–6.

[132] Pfeffer MA, Swedberg K, Granger CB, et al. Effects of candesartan on mortality and morbidity in patients with chronic heart failure: the CHARM-Overall programme. Lancet 2003;362(9386):759–66.

[133] Yusuf S, Sleight P, Pogue J, et al. Effects of an angiotensin-converting-enzyme inhibitor, ramipril, on cardiovascular events in high-risk patients. The Heart Outcomes Prevention Evaluation Study Investigators. N Engl J Med 2000;342(3):145–53.

[134] Major outcomes in high-risk hypertensive patients randomized to angiotensin-converting enzyme inhibitor or calcium channel blocker vs diuretic: The Antihypertensive and Lipid-Lowering Treatment to Prevent Heart Attack Trial (ALLHAT). JAMA 2002; 288(23):2981–97.

[135] Nesto RW, Bell D, Bonow RO, et al. Thiazolidinedione use, fluid retention, and congestive heart failure: a consensus statement for the American Heart Association and American Diabetes Association. Circulation 2003;108(23):2941–8.

[136] Attenuating insulin resistance as a therapeutic target in the management of heart failure. National Institutes of Health clinical research study (active). Bethesda (MD): US Department of Health, Education, and Welfare; 2005. NIH protocol # 03-H-0217.

ELSEVIER
SAUNDERS

Heart Failure Clin 2 (2006) 25 – 36

HEART
FAILURE
CLINICS

Diabetic Hypertension

Khurshid A. Khan, MD[a], Gurushankar Govindarajan, MD[b],
Adam Whaley-Connell, DO[a], James R. Sowers, MD[a],*

[a]University of Missouri–Columbia, Columbia, MO, USA
[b]Harry S. Truman Memorial Veterans Affairs Hospital, Columbia, MO, USA

Diabetes mellitus (DM) has become a worldwide epidemic. The prevalence of this chronic debilitating disease has increased dramatically over the past 40 years in the United States and worldwide. In 1985, there were approximately 30 million people who had DM worldwide; by the year 1995, this number had increased to 135 million [1]. According to current projections, the global incidence of DM in 2025 is expected to increase by 42%, bringing the total number of patients affected by DM to more than 300 million [2]. In addition to the recognized epidemic of DM in westernized cultures, the incidence of DM is also increasing in developing nations. By year 2025, more than 75% of people who have DM will reside in developing countries like India and China, compared with 62% in 1995 [2]. In the United States, at least 18 million people have been diagnosed as having DM; and an estimated 4 to 5 million remain undiagnosed. Based on national trends from 1980 to 1998, that number is expected to increase to 29 million by 2050 [3]. The epidemic of DM will continue to expand because of the growing prevalence of obesity in children [4]. In the last decade, the mean age at diagnosis of type 2 DM in the United States has decreased from 52 years to 46 years [5] and is now the leading cause of end-stage renal disease, new blindness, and nontraumatic amputations.

Cardiovascular disease (CVD) is the major cause of premature morbidity and mortality in patients who have type 2 DM. Coexistent hypertension accentuates the development of CVD and renal disease in these patients [6]. Complications associated with DM have increased along with the increase in prevalence of DM [7].

As the number of cases of DM increases, so will the socioeconomic impact. In 2002, the American Diabetes Association calculated the cost of DM to be $132 billion, or one out of every 10 dollars spent on health care in the United States [8]. Thus DM and related complications will consume increasingly more of health care resources.

Hypertension and diabetes

Currently, approximately 21 million people in the United States have been diagnosed as having DM, and an additional 65 million people are known to have hypertension. Hypertension frequently coexists with DM; the prevalence of hypertension in patients who have type 2 DM is up to three times greater than in age- and sex-matched patients who do not have DM [9,10]. Likewise, those patients who have documented hypertension are 2.5 times more prone to have diabetes than are their normotensive counterparts [11]. The coexistence of hypertension and DM markedly increases the development of CVD and chronic kidney disease (CKD) [12].

* Corresponding author. Division of Nephrology, Department of Internal Medicine, University of Missouri–Columbia, One Hospital Drive, MA410, DC043.00, Columbia, MO 65212.
E-mail address: sowersj@health.missouri.edu (J.R. Sowers).

1551-7136/06/$ – see front matter © 2006 Elsevier Inc. All rights reserved.
doi:10.1016/j.hfc.2005.11.002

heartfailure.theclinics.com

Cardiovascular disease in diabetes mellitus and hypertension

Hypertension and DM predispose to the development of CVD and CKD [12,13]. Persons who have DM are at about 60% increased risk for early mortality [12,14]. The age-adjusted relative risk for death caused by CVD events in persons who have type 2 DM is three-fold higher than in the general population. The presence of hypertension in patients who have DM substantially increases the risk for coronary heart disease, stroke, nephropathy, and retinopathy [15]. Indeed, when hypertension coexists with DM, the risk for CVD is increased by 75%, which further contributes to the overall morbidity and mortality of an already high-risk population [16]. Generally, hypertension in patients who have type 2 DM clusters with other CVD risk factors like microalbuminuria, central obesity, insulin resistance, dyslipidemia, hypercoagulation, increased inflammation, and left ventricular hypertrophy [9]. This clustering of risk factors in patients who have DM ultimately results in the development of CVD, which is the major cause of premature mortality in patients who have type 2 DM.

There is an increasing body of evidence from controlled clinical trials indicating that rigorous control of blood pressure (BP) to levels less than 130/80 mmHg markedly reduces CVD morbidity and mortality and the development of end-stage renal disease in persons who have type 2 DM [9]. A large population-based study in the United Kingdom demonstrated that the risk for a patient who has DM having myocardial infarction can be reduced by almost 10% for each reduction of systolic BP by 10 mmHg [17]. In recognition of this and other large randomized controlled clinical trials, the The Seventh Report of the Joint National Committee on Prevention, Detection, Evaluation, and Treatment of High Blood Pressure (JNC VII) noted that the risk for CVD events doubles for each incremental increase of 20 mmHg in systolic BP and 10 mmHg of diastolic BP starting at 115/75 mmHg [18]. CVD mortality in patients who have DM has been shown to decrease with aggressive management of BP and optimum treatment of other associated comorbid conditions, such as dyslipidemia and CKD [19,20].

Diabetic nephropathy in patients who have hypertension

The presence of diabetic nephropathy in conjunction with hypertension increases the risk for developing CKD and CVD. It is estimated that end-stage renal disease is increased five to six times in hypertensive patients who have DM compared with hypertensive patients who do not have DM [9,10]. Diabetic nephropathy has become the leading cause of end-stage renal disease in the United States [21,22]. Approximately 35% of persons who have DM will develop diabetic nephropathy, characterized by proteinuria, decreased glomerular filtration rate, and increased BP. Macroalbuminuria and microalbuminuria are major independent risk factors for CVD [23,24]. Indeed, microalbuminuria has been associated with insulin resistance, hyperinsulinemia, atherogenic dyslipidemia, and the absence of a nocturnal drop in systolic and diastolic BP, and has been identified as a part of the cardiometabolic syndrome [25]. In the Heart Outcomes Prevention Evaluation (HOPE) trial, the presence of albuminuria doubled the risk for the composite endpoint of myocardial infarction, stroke, or CVD death and all-cause mortality. The risk for heart failure was 3.7 times greater in type 2 DM patients who had microalbuminuria compared with those who did not. If current trends continue, approximately 175,000 new cases of end-stage renal disease will be diagnosed in 2010; and the Medicare cost of treatment will increase from $12 billion to $28 billion.

Stroke in patients who have diabetes and hypertension

Stroke is currently ranked as the third leading cause of death in the United States [26,27]. There are more than 700,000 strokes annually and more than 4.5 million stroke survivors. As the prevalence of DM increases, it has become a well-documented, independent, modifiable stroke risk factor [28]. Indeed, the incidence of stroke among DM patients is up to three times that in the general population [29]. There is an increase in short- and long-term mortality in patients who have DM following stroke. High admission glucose levels are one predictor of poor outcomes in these patients [28,29].

Hypertension in the cardiometabolic syndrome

The National Cholesterol Education Program Adult Treatment Panel III defines the cardiometabolic syndrome as presence of any three or more of the following: BP greater than or equal to 130/85 mmHg; waist circumference greater than 40 in for men and greater than 35 in for women; triglycerides greater than or equal to 150 mg/dL; high-density lipoprotein less than 40 mg/dL in men and less than 50 mg/dL in women; fasting glucose greater than or equal to

110 mg/dL. This syndrome is a clustering of maladaptive characteristics that confers an increased risk for CVD. The Framingham Heart Study demonstrated the synergistic action of these CVD risk factors in mediating CVD events. Indeed, the coexistence of hypertension, the cardiometabolic syndrome, or DM markedly increases the risk for developing macrovascular disease, which includes cerebrovascular, cardiovascular, and peripheral vascular diseases [30].

Pathophysiology of hypertension in the patient who has diabetes

Epidemiologic studies provide evidence for the coexistence of hypertension and DM and possibly point toward a common genetic and environmental factor promoting DM and hypertension. Similarly, clustering of hypertension, insulin resistance or type 2 DM, hyperlipidemia, and central obesity has also been documented in several populations [31]. Insulin resistance, increased tissue inflammation, increased reactive oxygen species production, endothelial dysfunction, increased tissue renin-angiotensin-aldosterone system (RAAS) activation, and increased sympathetic nervous system activity have all been implicated in this complex pathophysiology of DM and hypertension.

Insulin resistance

It is estimated that about 25% to 47% of persons who have hypertension also have insulin resistance or impaired glucose tolerance [31]. With insulin resistance, there are impaired biologic and physiologic tissue responses to insulin. Resistance to insulin, however, is not uniform in all tissues or for all insulin-signaling pathways. For example, the altered response of skeletal muscle and fat to insulin is accompanied by decreased insulin-mediated metabolic signaling and impaired glucose transport. Alternatively, accentuation of insulin growth effects with concurrent resistance to the metabolic actions gives rise to diverse clinical manifestations. The relationship among insulin resistance, DM, and hypertension is complex and interrelated. Untreated patients who have essential hypertension have higher fasting and postprandial insulin levels than age- and sex-matched normotensive persons, regardless of body mass; a direct correlation between plasma insulin levels and BP exists [32]. The relationship between hyperinsulinemia and hypertension is not seen in secondary hypertension [32], indicating that insulin resistance and hyperinsulinemia are not consequences of hypertension, but a genetic predisposition, which acts as a fertile soil for both diseases. This theory is supported by the observation that there is abnormal glucose metabolism in the offspring of hypertensive parents [33]. Thus, there is a strong association among hypertension, DM, and insulin resistance.

There is also a strong association among angiotensin II, hypertension, and DM [34,35]. It has been proposed that increased autocrine/paracrine activity of angiotensin II results in diminished phosphatidylinositol 3-kinase (PI3-K)- Akt signaling [36] and enhanced generation of reactive oxygen species, which may explain the impaired glucose use and hypertension associated with insulin resistance and type 2 DM [37]. Other possible causes of hypertension with insulin resistance/hyperinsulinemia include activation of the sympathetic nervous system, increased renal tubular sodium retention, elevated intracellular calcium concentration, vascular smooth muscle cell proliferation and atherosclerosis, impaired nitric oxide metabolism in skeletal muscle [38,39], and up-regulation of vascular angiotensin I receptors (AT_1R) by posttranscriptional mechanisms enhancing the vasoconstrictive and volume-expanding actions of the RAAS [40].

Vascular/endothelial dysfunction

Endothelial dysfunction is a key contributor to the development of hypertension and atherosclerosis and is associated with insulin resistance and obesity [41]. Insulin resistance and chronic hyperglycemia have been shown to cause endothelial dysfunction, leading to hypertension and diabetic nephropathy. Changes in vascular smooth muscle cells also contribute to hypertension in DM. Insulin exerts effects on endothelial cells and vascular smooth muscle cells by way of different mechanisms. In endothelial cells, insulin stimulates nitric oxide production through the PI3-K and Akt pathways [42] while it stimulates migration and growth of vascular smooth muscle cells by way of the mitogen-activated protein kinase pathway [43]. Defects in either or both of these pathways because of insulin resistance and hyperinsulinemia may result in the hypertension seen in patients with insulin-resistant and type 2 DM. In type 2 DM, nitric-oxide-dependent vasodilation is impaired because of an imbalance in production and inactivation. Superoxide dismutase, a free-radical scavenger, is suppressed in hypertension associated with DM. Moreover, plasma levels of asymmetric dimethylarginine, an endogenous competitive inhibitor of nitric oxide synthase, are significantly increased in hypertension associated with DM [44]. Collectively, these changes result in increased oxidative stress, formation of reactive oxygen species, and endothelial dysfunction that contribute to hypertension and CVD in patients who have DM.

DM is also associated with an increased generation of oxygen-derived free radicals, a source proposed to be the auto-oxidation of glucose. Oxygen-derived free radicals may impair endothelium-dependent vasodilatation through inactivation of nitric oxide [45]. Renal mesangial cells are thought to be modified vascular smooth muscle cells derived from the same progenitor mesenchymal cell line. Thus, the pathophysiologic alterations that cause endothelial dysfunction, leading to atherosclerosis and hypertension in DM, parallels the changes seen in diabetic glomerulosclerosis, resulting in proteinuria.

Sodium and volume retention

Alterations in sodium balance and extracellular fluid volume also play a role in the development of hypertension in DM. Insulin directly increases renal proximal tubular sodium reabsorption, having an antinatriuretic effect in normal, hypertensive, and insulin-resistant obese individuals [46]. In addition, suppression of atrial natriuretic peptide activity in the setting of hyperinsulinemia may also play a role in sodium retention in DM [47]. Sensitivity to dietary salt intake is greater in patients who are obese and have DM and low renin status, and contributes to sodium retention and extracellular fluid volume expansion. Thus, multiple mechanisms that contribute to hypertension and CVD may be involved in renal sodium handling and volume control in patients who have DM [48].

Increased sympathetic nervous system activity

Obesity-related hypertension is associated with increased sympathetic outflow to the kidneys as evidenced by increased renal vein noradrenaline levels [49]. There is also increased sympathetic activity to skeletal muscle vasculature as measured by microneurography. Leptin from adipose tissue, having important effects within the brain, may play a significant role in mediating the hypertension associated with obesity and the cardiometabolic syndrome. The high renal sympathetic tone likely contributes to the development of hypertension by stimulating renin secretion and promoting renal tubular reabsorption of sodium. Renal denervation in dogs has been shown to prevent sodium retention and hypertension associated with weight gain. Human studies have also demonstrated that increased plasma leptin levels in hypertensive individuals are associated with an increased heart rate and elevated plasma renin activity, angiotensinogen, and aldosterone levels, as well as hyperinsulinemia [50,51].

Renin-angiotensin-aldosterone system activation

Insulin is known to activate tissue RAAS [52]. Hypertension in DM is generally a low-renin, volume-expansion type of hypertension, which is often responsive to diuretic therapy. Furthermore, hypertension in DM is characterized by reduced nitric oxide–mediated vasorelaxation, reduced baroreflex sensitivity, and enhanced sympathetic nervous system activity, abnormalities that are promoted by aldosterone [45]. Changes in aldosterone secretion in response to changes in volume status or alteration in salt intake are mediated primarily by angiotensin II. Angiotensin II and aldosterone are known to exert genomic and nongenomic effects on the renal, systemic, and cerebral vasculature, resulting in adverse CVD outcomes [45]. There is increasing evidence that angiotensin II, acting through AT_1R, induces insulin resistance by inhibiting the actions of insulin in vascular and skeletal muscle tissue, in part, by interfering with insulin signaling through PI3-K and its downstream Akt signaling pathways [46]. Aldosterone also contributes to increases in fibrosis in the heart, the vasculature, and the kidney in patients with DM [45]. This notion is supported by emerging data that aldosterone antagonists improve cardiac diastolic dysfunction and vascular compliance, and reduce proteinuria in states of insulin resistance and type 2 DM [45]. RAAS activation may also contribute to promoting oxidative stress and endothelial dysfunction in DM [53]. Activation of RAAS is associated with increased nicotinamide adenosine dinucleotide plus hydrogen (NADH) and nicotinamide adenine dinucleotide phosphate (NADPH) oxidase activity and increased reactive oxygen species, such as the superoxide anion and hydrogen peroxide [54]. Interruption of RAAS by administration of angiotensin-converting enzyme (ACE) inhibitors or angiotensin receptor blockers (ARBs) improves insulin sensitivity and decreases the progression of type 2 DM in patients who are hypertensive [55].

Inflammation and oxidative stress

A chronic, low-level, inflammatory state often accompanies insulin resistance. Subclinical elevations of proinflammatory markers—interleukin-6, C-reactive protein associated with elevated white blood cell counts, plasminogen activator inhibitor-1, fibrinogen levels—are linked with the development of type 2 DM in adults [56]. This association is stronger in obese patients. Visceral fat accumulation is accompanied by progressive infiltration of macrophages [57], which secrete proinflammatory molecules, such as tumor necrosis factor α, interleukin 6, and interleukin 1β. These adipocytokines have been proposed to act through master proinflammatory regulators, such as those of the nuclear factor κB and the c-Jun NH2-terminal kinase (JNK)/AP-1 signaling pathways, to modulate the expression of genes coding for many inflammatory proteins and to alter insulin signaling. These actions have two basic consequences: first, to augment and perpetuate the proinflammatory diathesis, and second, to decrease insulin sensitivity [56]. Some adipocytokines have also been found to cause hypertension through direct pressor actions and interactions with the RAAS and the sympathetic nervous system [58].

Body composition and fat distribution

It has been proposed that angiotensin II has differential effects on the lipid storage capacity of adipose and skeletal muscle tissues such that muscle triglyceride accumulation occurs. This theory is supported by the resistance in patients who are abdominally obese and hypertensive to the antilipolytic actions of insulin, which is reversed by enalapril, and by decreased lipolysis in human skeletal muscle tissue with interstitial angiotensin II infusion. RAAS activity seems to effect the recruitment and differentiation of adipocytes; and recent studies suggest that ARBs may interact with the nuclear hormone receptor peroxisome proliferator-activated receptor γ (PPAR-γ) independent of AT$_1$R. PPAR-γ is the cellular target for the insulin-sensitizing thiazolidinedione drugs, and therefore ARB interaction may represent a potential mechanism by which ARBs improve insulin sensitivity. Furthermore, increases in plasma adiponectin have been reported with either an ACE inhibitor (temocapril) or ARB (candesartan). Adiponectin is the adipocytokine produced in greatest abundance, but circulating levels are decreased with obesity. Adiponectin administration has been shown to improve insulin action in animals, while low levels of adiponectin are proposed to contribute to obesity associated insulin resistance.

Management

There is overwhelming evidence that reduction of BP in DM decreases CVD mortality and the progression of CKD. Clinical trials in patients who are hypertensive have shown that the reduction of BP decreases the incidence of stroke by 35% to 40%, myocardial infarction by 20% to 25%, and heart failure by 50% [59]. The JNC VII recommends a goal BP of less than 130/80 mmHg in patients who have DM and CKD [59]. This goal BP is also supported by the World Health Organization, International Society of Hypertension, and the National Kidney Foundation [60,61].

The Hypertension Optimal Treatment (HOT) trial demonstrated that patients who had DM had a 51% reduction of risk in CVD events when their diastolic BP target was less than 80 mmHg, when compared with those whose target was less than 90 mmHg [62]. Epidemiologic analysis of the data from the United Kingdom Prospective Diabetes Study (UKPDS) cohort also shows a linear relationship between CVD risk and systolic BP starting at 120 mmHg and above [63]. In addition, results from the Systolic Hypertension in the Elderly Program (SHEP) and Systolic Hypertension in Europe (Syst-Eur) trials also favor the aggressive antihypertensive treatment of patients who have DM with isolated systolic hypertension [64]. A recent survey, using the Framingham algorithm to evaluate coronary risk in individuals in the third National Health and Nutrition Examination Survey (NHANES III) who have the cardiometabolic syndrome, estimated that controlling BP to normal levels (120–129/80–84 mmHg) would prevent 28.1% of coronary events in men and 12.5% of events in women [65].

Nonpharmacologic treatment

The current recommendation of the JNC VII emphasizes the need for the adoption of a healthy lifestyle for the prevention and treatment of hypertension. Indeed, aggressive nonpharmacologic interventions are pivotal and indispensable in the therapeutic outcome in all hypertensive populations.

Weight loss

Several randomized controlled trials have documented the value of modest weight loss in decreasing the risk for hypertension [66]. The main strategies used to implement weight loss are diet and exercise. A loss of 10 kg weight is associated with decrease in systolic BP of 5 to 20 mmHg.

Diet

The Dietary Approaches to Stop Hypertension (DASH) Study, a diet rich in fruits, vegetables, and low-fat dairy products, with a reduced content of saturated fat and total fat, has been proved to reduce systolic BP by 8 to14 mmHg, significantly more in people who are hypertensive than in those who are normotensive [67]. In addition to improving glycemic control, a diet that is high in fiber and potassium and lower in saturated fats, refined carbohydrates, and salt can improve the lipid profile and significantly lower blood pressure [68]. Dietary sodium reduction of less than 100 mmol/d can lower systolic BP by 2 to 8 mmHg.

Exercise

Physical activity is also beneficial for lowering BP and improving insulin sensitivity. The Finnish Diabetes Prevention Study showed that intensified lifestyle intervention, consisting of diet and moderate exercise for at least 30 minutes per day, in overweight subjects who were glucose-intolerant resulted not only in a marked reduction in the risk for developing type 2 DM, but also in a significant drop in BP (4 mmHg for systolic BP and 2 mmHg for diastolic BP compared with control subjects) [69]. A prospective study of 8302 Finnish men and 9139 women showed that regular physical activity was associated with a significantly reduced risk for hypertension in men and women, independent of age, education, smoking habits, alcohol intake, history of DM, body mass index, and systolic BP at baseline [70]. Overweight and obesity were also associated with an increased risk for hypertension; and the protective effect of physical activity was consistent in overweight and normal weight subjects. Most of the studies have shown that the most benefit is derived from aerobic exercise [71]. Data on effects of the intensity of physical activity on hypertension, however, are conflicting. The most recent data demonstrates that high physical activity, defined as a combination of vigorous occupational activity more than 30 minutes daily and leisure-time physical activity more than 4 hours a week, is associated with a lower risk for hypertension, independent of baseline body mass index [70].

Other factors

Lastly, patients should be counseled on smoking cessation to reduce their overall CVD risk. It is also important to limit consumption of alcohol to no more than two drinks per day for men and to no more than one drink per day in women and lightweight persons.

Pharmacotherapy

The JNC VII recommendations are consistent with guidelines from the American Diabetes Association, National Kidney Foundation, World Health Organization, and International Society of Hypertension, which has also recommend that BP in people with DM be controlled to levels of less than 130/80 mmHg [72]. Whatever the goal level, rigorous control of BP is paramount for reducing CVD mortality and morbidity [72]. Achieving goal BP in patients who have DM usually requires two or more drugs [73]. There is convincing evidence regarding certain classes of drugs that seem to offer certain beneficial effects over others in patients who have hypertensive diabetics.

ACE inhibitors

The RAAS plays a role in almost every step in the progression of atherosclerosis and hypertension. Multiple clinical trials have demonstrated the pleiotropic effects of the ACE inhibitors. In addition to being an effective antihypertensive, ACE inhibitors have been proved to offer additional benefits in patients who have DM. The HOPE trial studied 9541 patients, 3577 of whom had DM. Ramipril use was associated with a significant 25% risk reduction in myocardial infarction, stroke, or cardiovascular death after a median follow-up period of 4.5 years [74]. This benefit was independent of any BP-lowering effect. Furthermore, the microalbuminuric, cardiovascular, and renal outcomes in the HOPE substudy (MICRO-HOPE) also showed that ramipril treatment was associated with a decreased risk for development of overt nephropathy in patients who had type 2 DM with microalbuminuria [75].

Of the 10,985 patients in the Captopril Prevention Project (CAPP), 309 patients in the captopril group and 263 in the conventional therapy group had DM. Overall, captopril treatment markedly lowered the risk for fatal and nonfatal myocardial infarction, stroke, and cardiovascular deaths, more than the beta-blocker or diuretic therapy used in the conventional therapy group [76]. The effects of the two regimens in the diabetic subpopulation showed a clear difference in the risk for developing a primary endpoint in favor of a captopril-based regimen [77,78].

In addition to lowering the BP, ACE inhibitors decrease membrane permeability to albumin and intraglomerular pressure. By reducing microalbuminuria,

ACE inhibitors can help prevent the progression of diabetic nephropathy. Meta-analyses have shown that this antiproteinuric effect is independent of the changes in BP. ACE inhibitors have also been shown to slow the progression of diabetic nephropathy in microalbuminuric, normotensive patients compared with other antihypertensives. Renal function should be carefully monitored after initiation of ACE inhibitor therapy. Although a slight increase in serum creatinine may be expected, an increase of more than 30% or a continual increase during the first two months of therapy should raise suspicion about the possibility of renal artery stenosis or significant volume depletion [60]. Volume depletion is an important cause for the increase in creatinine initially and is often correctable.

There is also increasing data suggesting that these agents have direct effects on improving insulin sensitivity [74–76]. A 14% reduction in the risk for new onset DM was observed in the CAPP trial compared with conventional therapy with either a beta blocker, diuretic or both. A 34% relative risk reduction for developing DM was also observed in the HOPE trial. The Diabetic Reduction Approaches With Ramipril and Rosiglitazone Medications (DREAM), a randomized, controlled clinical trial, is currently evaluating the effect of ramipril, rosiglitazone, or a combination of both versus placebo in preventing the progression from insulin resistance or the cardiometabolic syndrome to type 2 DM.

Angiotensin receptor blockers

Other medications receiving considerable attention in recent years are the ARBs. Antihypertensive actions of ARBs are roughly equivalent to those of ACE inhibitors, but ARBs do have an improved side-effect profile when compared with ACE inhibitors. Like ACE inhibitors, ARBs have similar beneficial effects in reducing the progression of diabetic nephropathy and improving cardiovascular and renal outcomes, by virtue of their RAAS blockade [82]. Several clinical trials demonstrate that ARBs also have beneficial effects on glucose metabolism that are likely independent of bradykinin-mediated mechanisms [79–82]. In the Losartan Intervention For Endpoint reduction in hypertension (LIFE) study, losartan reduced the relative risk for developing type 2 DM by 25% when compared with the beta blocker atenolol. In the absence of a placebo control group in the study, however, it is possible that the reduction in incidence of DM could reflect the net result of increased insulin sensitivity in the losartan group and increased insulin resistance in the atenolol group [81]. Similarly, reduction in the relative risk for

developing DM was noted in the Candesartan in Heart failure: Assessment of Reduction in Mortality and morbidity (CHARM) studies [80,82]. The Valsartan Antihypertensive Long-Term Use Evaluation (VALUE) trial demonstrated the advantage of an ARB, valsartan, over a calcium channel blocker, amlodipine, in reducing the relative risk for new-onset DM by 23% in patients aged 50 years or older who had hypertension [83].

ACE inhibitor/ARB studies so far assessed the incidence of type 2 DM as a secondary endpoint. The consistent and promising findings noted from these studies resulted in the initiation of studies to clarify the extent by which the inhibition of RAAS can reduce the incidence of new-onset DM. The DREAM trial is a large, international, multi-center, randomized, prospective double-blind controlled trial involving 4000 people, randomized to receive either ramipril or rosiglitazone using a 2×2 factorial design and assessed for new-onset DM [84]. The Nateglinide And Valsartan in Impaired Glucose Tolerance Outcomes Research (NAVIGATOR) study is evaluating the effects of an oral antidiabetic drug, nateglinide, and an ARB, valsartan, on prevention of type 2 DM in patients who have impaired glucose tolerance. This study is similar to DREAM, but is a larger trial than DREAM (7500 subjects compared with 4000) and also investigates the effects of antidiabetic/antihypertensive therapy on the development of CVD in people who have impaired glucose tolerance [85].

Collectively, these ongoing studies are expected to clarify the extent by which inhibition of the RAAS can reduce the incidence of new onset DM in patients who have impaired glucose tolerance, a group that includes many Americans who have essential hypertension [86].

Beta blockers

Beta blockers can be effective antihypertensive agents in the diabetic population as part of a multi-drug regimen. Beta-blockade also finds its use in DM patients who have concomitant evidence of coronary artery disease, such as anginal symptoms, including anginal equivalents, or postmyocardial infarction. The effectiveness of beta blockers was demonstrated in the UKPDS in that atenolol was comparable to captopril in reduction of CVD outcomes [87,88]. Although these agents have been associated with adverse effects on glucose and lipid profiles and implicated in new-onset DM in obese patients, they are not absolutely contraindicated for use in patients who have DM. In fact, carvedilol, which has α- and β-receptor blocking properties, has been shown to induce vasodilatation and improve insulin sensitivity [89]. Also, in The Glycemic Effects in Diabetes Mellitus: Carvedilol-Metoprolol Comparison in Hypertensive [GEMINI]) study showed that carvedilol in the presence of RAAS blockade is superior to metaprolol in improving some of the metabolic complication associated with DM, including microalbuminuria, without affecting the glycemic control [87].

Thiazide diuretics

Thiazides have been shown to cause electrolyte imbalances, metabolic changes, and volume contraction. Nevertheless, in the Antihypertensive and Lipid-Lowering treatment to prevent Heart Attack Trial (ALLHAT), which compared a thiazide (chlorthalidone) to a calcium channel blocker (amlodipine) or an ACE inhibitor (lisinopril), found that the thiazide was less expensive and superior to the ACE inhibitor or calcium channel blocker in lowering the incidence of CVD in hypertensive populations [90]. Therefore, ALLHAT suggests that thiazides could be considered as a first-line therapy for many diabetic patients who have hypertension [90], even though they may adversely affect insulin resistance and potassium balance in some individuals. Indeed, using a thiazide diuretic in the antihypertensive repertoire has been shown consistently to improve CVD outcomes, even in those who have DM [91]. Treating volume expansion with thiazide diuretics can increase the activity of the RAAS. Thus, combining a diuretic with an ACE inhibitor, or an ARB, can be an effective BP-lowering combination.

Calcium channel blockers

It has been shown in that nondihydropyridine calcium channel blockers, such as verapamil and diltiazem, decrease proteinuria in patients who have DM [73]. Not to the degree of ACE inhibitors alone, but in combination therapy, nondihydropyridine calcium channel blockers and ACE inhibitors have been shown to have the additive effect of reducing albuminuria [92]. The Syst-Eur trial with nitrendipine demonstrated that intensive antihypertensive therapy for older patients who had type 2 DM and isolated systolic hypertension eliminated the additional risk for CVD events and stroke associated with diabetes [93]. In the HOT trial, there was a reduction in major CVD events with diastolic BP control in patients who had DM, when felodipine was used as first-line therapy [94]. Thus, calcium channel blockers are not harmful or contraindicated in hypertensive patients who have diabetes; and the combination of an ACE inhibitor and a calcium antagonist is effective for the management of hypertension in patients who have DM [95].

Others

Hydralazine, a direct-acting vasodilator, can also be recommended for patients who have coexistent systolic heart failure and hypertension, who cannot tolerate an ACE inhibitor or ARB, or have contraindications to the above agents [96].

Clonidine, an alpha-2 agonist, can be helpful in treating patients who have supine hypertension associated with orthostatic hypotension; but its use is limited by side effects that primarily include central nervous system effects, sexual dysfunction, and dry mouth. Alpha-2 agonists do not have adverse lipid effects, but do have the potential to inhibit pancreatic beta-cell insulin secretion, thereby impairing glucose metabolism [97].

Summary

DM is a growing epidemic in the developing and developed world. It places an enormous socioeconomic burden on already sparse resources. Patients who have DM have a higher risk for development of hypertension and subsequent CVD and CKD. Patients who have DM and hypertension present a special challenge to clinicians, and an individualized approach should be used in management. Quality of life, adverse effects of anti-hypertensive medications, and other comorbid conditions all play a role in the successful management of hypertension. The presence of peripheral vascular disease, congestive heart failure, coronary artery disease, orthostatic hypotension, dyslipidemia, and diabetic nephropathy all influence the choice of agent. More important is for the physician and his or her health care team to work closely with each individual patient to attain, prudently but aggressively, the goal BP of less than 130/80 mmHg.

References

[1] International Diabetes Federation Task Force on Diabetes Health Economics. Facts, Figures and Forecasts. Brussels (Belguim): International Diabetes Federation; 1997.

[2] King H, Aubert RE, Herman WH. Global burden of diabetes, 1995–2025: prevalence, numerical estimates, and projections. Diabetes Care 1998;21(9):1414–31.

[3] Winer N, Sowers JR. Epidemiology of diabetes. J Clin Pharmacol 2004;44(4):397–405.

[4] Pinhas-Hamiel O, Zeitler P. The global spread of type 2

diabetes mellitus in children and adolescents. J Pediatr 2005;146(5):693–700.

[5] Koopman RJ, Mainous III AG, Diaz VA, et al. Changes in age at diagnosis of type 2 diabetes mellitus in the United States, 1988 to 2000. Ann Fam Med 2005;3(1):60–3.

[6] Department of Health and Human Services, Centers for Disease Control and Prevention. National Diabetes Fact Sheet. General information and national estimates on diabetes in the United States. 2003.

[7] Bakris G, Williams M, Dworkin L, et al. Preserving renal function in adults with hypertension and diabetes: a consensus approach. Am J Kidney Dis 2000;36(3): 646–61.

[8] Economic costs of diabetes in the US in 2002. Diabetes Care 2003;26(3):917–32.

[9] Sowers JR, Epstein M, Frolich ED. Diabetes, hypertension, and cardiovascular disease: an update. Hypertension 2001;37:1053–9.

[10] Sowers JR, Williams M, Epstein M, et al. Hypertension in patients with diabetes: strategies for drug therapy to reduce complications. Postgrad Med 2000; 107:47–54.

[11] Gress TW, Nieto FJ, Shahar E, et al. Hypertension and antihypertensive therapy as risk factors for type 2 diabetes mellitus. N Engl J Med 2000;342:905–12.

[12] El-Atat F, McFarlane SI, Sowers JR. Diabetes, hypertension, and cardiovascular derangements: pathophysiology and management. Curr Hypertens Rep 2004;6: 215–23.

[13] Sowers JR. Treatment of hypertension in patients with diabetes. Arch Intern Med 2004;164:1850–7.

[14] Miettinen H, Lehto S, Salomaa V, et al. Impact of diabetes on mortality after the first myocardial infarction. The FINMONICA Myocardial Infarction Register Study Group. Diabetes Care 1998;21(1):69–75.

[15] Sowers JR, Haffner S. Treatment of cardiovascular and renal risk factors in the diabetic hypertensive. Hypertension 2002;40(6):781–8.

[16] Adler AI, Stratton IM, Neil HAW, et al. Association of systolic blood pressure with macrovascular and microvascular complications of type 2 diabetes (UKPDS 36): prospective observational study. BMJ 2000; 321(7258):412–9.

[17] Position Statement American Diabetes Association. Treatment of hypertension in adults with diabetes. Diabetes Care 2002;25:71S–3S.

[18] Chobanian AV, Bakris GL, Black HR, et al. The seventh report of the Joint National Committee on Prevention, Detection, Evaluation, and Treatment of High Blood Pressure: The JNC 7 Report. JAMA 2003; 289(19):2560–71.

[19] McFarlane SI, Jacober SJ, Winer N, et al. Control of cardiovascular risk factors in patients with diabetes and hypertension at urban academic medical centers. Diabetes Care 2002;25(4):718–23.

[20] Sowers JR. Recommendations for special populations: diabetes mellitus and the metabolic syndrome. Am J Hypertens 2003;16(11 Pt 2):41S–5S.

[21] Tuomilehto J, Lindstrom J, Eriksson JG, et al, Finnish Diabetes Prevention Study Group. Prevention of type 2 diabetes mellitus by changes in lifestyle among subjects with impaired glucose tolerance. N Engl J Med 2001;344:1343–50.

[22] Sacks FM, Svetkey LP, Vollmer WM, et al, DASH Sodium Collaborative Research Group. Effects on blood pressure of reduced dietary sodium and the Dietary Approaches to Stop Hypertension (DASH) diet. N Engl J Med 2001;344:3–10.

[23] Eknoyan G, Hostetter T, Bakris GL, et al. Proteinuria and other markers of chronic kidney disease: a position statement of the National Kidney Foundation (NKF) and the national institute of Diabetes and digestive and kidney diseases (NIDDK). Am J Kidney Dis 2003;42: 617–22.

[24] Dineen SF, Gerstein HC. The association of microalbuminuria and mortality in non-insulin-dependent diabetes mellitus: a systematic overview of the literature. Arch Intern Med 1997;157:1413–8.

[25] Jensen JS, Feldt-Rusmussen B, Strandgaard S, et al. Arterial hypertension, microalbuminuria, and risk of ischemic heart disease. Hypertension 2000;35:898–903.

[26] Goldstein LB, Adams R, Becker K, et al. Primary prevention of ischemic stroke: a statement for healthcare professionals from the stroke council of the American Heart Association. Circulation 2001;103: 163–82.

[27] Tuomilchte J, Rastenyte D. Diabetes and glucose intolerance as risk factors for stroke. J Cardiovasc Risk 1999;6:241–9.

[28] Bell DSH. Stroke in the diabetic patient. Diabetes Care 1994;17:213–9.

[29] Sacco RL. Reducing the risk of stroke in diabetes: what have we learned that is new? Diabetes Obes Metab 2002;4(Suppl 1):S27–34.

[30] National diabetes fact sheet. General information and national estimates on diabetes in the United States 2003.

[31] Reaven GM. Banting lecture 1988. Role of insulin resistance in human disease. Diabetes 1988;37(12): 1595–607.

[32] Sechi LA, Melis A, Tedde R. Insulin hypersecretion: a distinctive feature between essential and secondary hypertension. Metabolism 1992;41(11):1261–6.

[33] Sowers JR, Bakris GL. Antihypertensive therapy and the risk of type 2 diabetes mellitus. N Engl J Med 2000;342(13):969–70.

[34] Richey JM, Ader M, Moore D, et al. Angiotensin II induces insulin resistance independent of changes in interstitial insulin. Am J Physiol Endocrinol Metab 1999;277(5):E920–6.

[35] Ogihara T, Asano T, Ando K, et al. Angiotensin ii–induced insulin resistance is associated with enhanced insulin signaling. Hypertension 2002;40(6):872–9.

[36] Sloniger JA, Saengsirisuwan V, Diehl CJ, et al. Defective insulin signaling in skeletal muscle of the hypertensive TG(mREN2)27 rat. Am J Physiol Endocrinol Metab 2005;288(6):E1074–81.

[37] Sowers JR. Insulin resistance and hypertension. Am J Physiol Heart Circ Physiol 2004;286(5):H1597–602.

[38] Modan M, Halkin H. Hyperinsulinemia or increased sympathetic drive as links for obesity and hypertension. Diabetes Care 1991;14(6):470–87.

[39] DeFronzo RA, Ferrannini E. Insulin resistance. A multifaceted syndrome responsible for NIDDM, obesity, hypertension, dyslipidemia, and atherosclerotic cardiovascular disease. Diabetes Care 1991;14(3):173–94.

[40] Nickenig G, Roling J, Strehlow K, et al. Insulin induces upregulation of vascular AT1 receptor gene expression by posttranscriptional mechanisms. Circulation 1998;98(22):2453–60.

[41] Caballero AE. Endothelial dysfunction in obesity and insulin resistance: a road to diabetes and heart disease. Obes Res 2003;11:1278–89.

[42] Kuboki K, Jiang ZY, Takahara N, et al. Regulation of endothelial constitutive nitric oxide synthase gene expression in endothelial cells in vivo: a specific vascular action of insulin. Circulation 2000;101: 676–81.

[43] Hsueh WA, Quinones M. Role of endothelial dysfunction in insulin resistance. Am J Cardiol 2003; 92(Suppl):10J–7J.

[44] Williams SB, Cusco JA, Roddy MA, et al. Impaired nitric oxide-mediated vasodilation in patients with non-insulin-dependent diabetes mellitus. J Am Coll Cardiol 1996;27:567–74.

[45] McFarlane SI, Sowers JR. Aldosterone function in diabetes mellitus: effects on cardiovascular and renal disease. J Clin Endocrinol Metab 2003;88:516–23.

[46] Sowers JR, Sowers PS, Peuler JD. Role of insulin resistance and hyperinsulinemia in development of hypertension and atherosclerosis. J Lab Clin Med 1994;123:647–52.

[47] Feldt-Rasmussen B, Mathiesen ER, Deckert T, et al. Central role for sodium in the pathogenesis of blood pressure changes independent of angiotensin, aldosterone and catecholamines in type 1 (insulin-dependent) diabetes mellitus. Diabetologia 1987;30:610–7.

[48] Sowers JR. Effects of insulin and IGF-I on vascular smooth muscle glucose and cation metabolism. Diabetes 1996;45:S47–51.

[49] Fagan TC, Sowers J. Type 2 diabetes mellitus: greater cardiovascular risks and greater benefits of therapy. Arch Intern Med 1999;159:1033–4.

[50] Facchini F, Chen Y-DI, Clinkingbeard C, et al. Insulin resistance, hyperinsulinemia, and dyslipidemia in non-obese individuals with a family history of hypertension. Am J Hypertens 1992;5:694–9.

[51] Reaven GM, Lithell H, Landsberg L. Hypertension and associated metabolic abnormalities: the role of insulin resistance and the sympathoadrenal system. N Engl J Med 1996;334:374–82.

[52] DeFronzo RA, Ferrannini E. Insulin resistance: a multifaceted syndrome responsible for NIDDM, obesity, hypertension, dyslipidemia and atherosclerotic cardiovascular disease. Diabetes Care 1991;14:173–94.

[53] Sowers JR, Haffner S. Treatment of cardiovascular and renal risk factors in the diabetic hypertensive. Hypertension 2002;40:781–8.

[54] Dzau VJ. Theodore Cooper Lecture: tissue angiotensin and pathobiology of vascular disease: a unifying hypothesis. Hypertension 2001;37:1047–52.

[55] McFarlane SI, Kumar A, Sowers JR. Mechanisms by which angiotensin-converting enzyme inhibitors prevent diabetes and cardiovascular disease. Am J Cardiol 2003;91:30H–7H.

[56] Duncan BB, Schmidt MI, Pankow JS, et al. Low-grade systemic inflammation and the development of diabetes: The Atherosclerosis Risk in Communities Study. Diabetes 2003;52:1799–805.

[57] Weisberg SP, McCann D, Desnai M, et al. Obesity is associated with macrophage accumulation in adipose tissue. J Clin Invest 2003;112:1796–808.

[58] Fernández-Real JM, Ricart W. Insulin resistance and chronic cardiovascular inflammatory syndrome. Endocr Rev 2003;24(3):278–301.

[59] Chobanian AV, Bakris GL, Black HR, et al. Seventh report of the Joint National Committee on Prevention, Detection, Evaluation, and Treatment of High Blood Pressure. JAMA 2003;289(19):2560–71.

[60] Bakris GL, Williams M, Dworkin L, et al. Preserving renal function in adults with hypertension and diabetes: a consensus approach. National Kidney Foundation Hypertension and Diabetes Executive Committees Working Group. Am J Kidney Dis 2000;36:646–61.

[61] World Health Organization/International Society of Hypertension Writing Group. 2003 World Health Organization (WHO)/International Society of Hypertension (ISH) statement on management of hypertension. J Hypertens 2003;21(11):1983–92.

[62] Hansson L, Zanchetti A, Carruthers SG, et al. Effects of intensive blood pressure lowering and low-dose aspirin in patients with hypertension: principal results of the Hypertension Optimal Treatment (HOT) randomized trial. Lancet 1998;351:1755–62.

[63] Adler AI, Stratton IM, Neil HAW, et al on behalf of the UK Prospective Diabetes Study Group. Association of systolic blood pressure with macrovascular and microvascular complications of type 2 diabetes (UKPDS 36): prospective observational study. BMJ 2000;321: 412–9.

[64] Curb JD, Pressel SL, Cutler J, et al. Effect of diuretic-based antihypertensive treatment on cardiovascular risk in older diabetic patients with isolated systolic hypertension. JAMA 1996;276:1886–92.

[65] Wong ND, Pio JR, Franklin SS, et al. Preventing coronary events by optimal control of blood pressure and lipids in patients with the metabolic syndrome. Am J Cardiol 2003;91(12):1421–6.

[66] Trials of Hypertension Prevention Collaborative Research Group. The effects of nonpharmacologic interventions on blood pressure of persons with high normal levels: results of the Trials of Hypertension Prevention Phase 1. JAMA 1992;267:1213–20.

[67] He J, Whelton PK, Appel LJ, et al. Long-term effects of weight loss and dietary sodium reduction on

incidence of hypertension. Hypertension 2000;35: 544–9.

[68] Wassertheil-Smoller S, Blaufox D, Oberman AS, et al. The Trial of Antihypertensive Interventions and Management (TAIM) Study: Adequate weight loss, alone and combined with drug therapy in the treatment of mild hypertension. Arch Intern Med 1992;152: 131–6.

[69] Tuomilehto J, Lindstrom J, Eriksson JG, et al. Prevention of type 2 diabetes mellitus by changes in lifestyle among subjects with impaired glucose tolerance. N Engl J Med 2001;344:1343–50.

[70] Hu G, Barengo NC, Tuomilehto J, et al. Relationship of physical activity and body mass index to the risk of hypertension: A prospective study in Finland. Hypertension 2004;43:25–30.

[71] Whelton SP, Chin A, Xin X, et al. Effect of aerobic exercise on blood pressure: a meta-analysis of randomized, controlled trials. Ann Intern Med 2002;136: 493–503.

[72] Whaley-Connell A, Sowers JR. Hypertension management in type 2 diabetes mellitus: recommendations of the Joint National Committee VII. Endocrinol Metab Clin N Am 2005;34(1):63–75.

[73] Arauz-Pacheco C, Parrott MA, Raskin P. The treatment of hypertension in adult patients with diabetes. Diabetes Care 2002;25(1):134–47.

[74] Yosuf S, Sleight P, Pogue J, et al. Effects of an angiotensin-converting-enzyme inhibitor, ramipril, on cardiovascular events in high-risk patients. The Heart Outcomes Prevention Evaluation Study Investigators. N Engl J Med 2000;342:145–53.

[75] Heart Outcomes Prevention Evaluation Study Investigators. Effects of ramipril on cardiovascular and microvascular outcomes in people with diabetes mellitus: results of the HOPE study and MICRO-HOPE substudy. Lancet 2000;355:253–9.

[76] Hansson L, Lindholm LH, Niskanen L, et al for the Captopril Prevention Project (CAPPP) study group. Effect of angiotensin-converting-enzyme inhibition compared with conventional morbidity and mortality in hypertension: the Captopril Prevention Project (CAPPP) randomised trial. Lancet 1999;353:611–6.

[77] Niskanen L, Hedner T, Hansson L, et al. Reduced cardiovascular morbidity and mortality in hypertensive diabetic patients on first-line therapy with an ACE inhibitor compared with a diuretic/β-blocker–based treatment regimen: A subanalysis of the Captopril Prevention Project. Diabetes Care 2001;24:2091–6.

[78] Scheen AJ. Renin-angiotensin system inhibition prevents type 2 diabetes mellitus. Part 1. Meta-analysis of randomised clinical trials. Diabetes Metab 2004;30(6): 487–96.

[79] Lindholm LH, Persson M, Alaupovic P, et al. Metabolic outcome during 1 year in newly detected hypertensives: results of the Antihypertensive Treatment and Lipid Profile in a North of Sweden Efficacy Evaluation (ALPINE study). J Hypertens 2003;21(8): 1563–74.

[80] Pfeffer MA, Swedberg K, Granger CB, et al. Effects of candesartan on mortality and morbidity in patients with chronic heart failure: the CHARM-Overall programme. Lancet 2003;362:759–66.

[81] Lindholm LH, Ibsen H, Borch-Johnsen K, et al. Risk of new-onset diabetes in the Losartan Intervention For Endpoint reduction in hypertension study. J Hypertens 2002;20(9):1879–86.

[82] Yusuf S, Pfeffer MA, Swedberg K, et al. Effects of candesartan in patients with chronic heart failure and preserved left-ventricular ejection fraction: the CHARM-Preserved Trial. Lancet 2003;362:777–81.

[83] Julius S, Kjeldsen SE, Weber M, et al. Outcomes in hypertensive patients at high cardiovascular risk treated with regimens based on valsartan or amlodipine: the VALUE randomised trial. Lancet 2004;363: 2022–31.

[84] Gerstein HC, Yusuf S, Holman R, et al. Rationale, design and recruitment characteristics of a large, simple international trial of diabetes prevention: the DREAM trial. Diabetologia 2004;47(9):1519–27.

[85] Califf RM. Insulin resistance: a global epidemic in need of effective therapies. Eur Heart J 2003;5(Suppl C): C13–8.

[86] Scheen AJ. Prevention of type 2 diabetes mellitus through inhibition of the renin-angiotensin system. Drugs 2004;64(22):2537–65.

[87] Bakris GL, et al. Metabolic effects of carvedilol vs metoprolol in patients with type 2 diabetes mellitus and hypertension: a randomized controlled trial. JAMA 2004;292:2227–36.

[88] Group UKPDS. Tight blood pressure control and risk of macrovascular and microvascular complications in type 2 diabetes: UKPDS 38. BMJ 1998;317(7160): 703–13.

[89] Group UKPDS. Efficacy of atenolol and captopril in reducing risk of macrovascular and microvascular complications in type 2 diabetes: UKPDS 39. BMJ 1998; 317(7160):713–20.

[90] Giugliano D, Acampora R, Marfella R, et al. Metabolic and Cardiovascular Effects of Carvedilol and Atenolol in Non-Insulin-Dependent Diabetes Mellitus and Hypertension: a randomized, controlled trial. Ann Intern Med 1997;126(12):955–9.

[91] Major outcomes in high-risk hypertensive patients randomized to angiotensin-converting enzyme inhibitor or calcium channel blocker vs diuretic: The Antihypertensive and Lipid-Lowering Treatment to Prevent Heart Attack Trial (ALLHAT). JAMA 2002;288(23): 2981–97.

[92] Curb JD, Pressel SL, Cutler JA, et al. Effect of diuretic-based antihypertensive treatment on cardiovascular disease risk in older diabetic patients with isolated systolic hypertension. Systolic Hypertension in the Elderly Program Cooperative Research Group. JAMA 1996;276(23):1886–92.

[93] Bakris GL, Smith AC, Richardson DJ, et al. Impact of an ACE inhibitor and calcium antagonist on micro-albuminuria and lipid subfractions in type 2 diabetes: a

randomised, multi-centre pilot study. J Hum Hypertens 2002;16(3):185–91.

[94] Birkenhager WH, Staessen JA, Gasowski J, et al. Effects of antihypertensive treatment on endpoints in the diabetic patients randomized in the Systolic Hypertension in Europe (Syst-Eur) trial. J Nephrol 2000; 13(3):232–7.

[95] Hansson L, Zanchetti A, Carruthers SG, et al. Effects of intensive blood-pressure lowering and low-dose aspirin in patients with hypertension: principal results of the Hypertension Optimal Treatment (HOT) randomised trial. HOT Study Group. Lancet 1998;351: 1755–62.

[96] Poulter NR. Calcium antagonists and the diabetic patient: a response to recent controversies. Am J Cardiol 1998;82(9B):40R–1R.

[97] Hunt SA, Baker DW, Chin MH, et al. ACC/AHA guidelines for the evaluation and management of chronic heart failure in the adult: executive summary. A report of the American College of Cardiology/ American Heart Association task force on practice guidelines (committee to revise the 1995 guidelines for the evaluation and management of heart failure) developed in collaboration with the International Society for Heart and Lung Transplantation endorsed by the Heart Failure Society of America. J Am Coll Cardiol 2001;38:2101.

Further readings

Leclercq-Meyer V, Herchuelz A, Valverde I, et al. Mode of action of clonidine upon islet function: dissociated effects upon the time course and magnitude of insulin release. Diabetes 1980;29:193–200.

Lind L, Berne C, Lithell H. Prevalence of insulin resistance in essential hypertension. J Hypertens 1995;13:1457–62.

Sowers JR. Insulin and insulin-like growth factor in normal and pathological cardiovascular physiology. Hypertension 1997;29:691–9.

Weinberger MH. Salt sensitive human hypertension. Endocr Res 1991;17:43–51.

ELSEVIER
SAUNDERS

Heart Failure Clin 2 (2006) 37 – 52

HEART
FAILURE
CLINICS

Diabetic Dyslipidemia and the Heart

Abu R. Vasudevan, MBBS, MD, MRCP(UK)[a], Alan J. Garber, MD, PhD[b],*

[a]Center for Cadiovascular Disease Prevention, Lipoprotein and Atherosclerosis Research Section,
Baylor College of Medicine, Houston, TX, USA
[b]Division of Endocrinology and Molecular and Cell Biology, Baylor College of Medicine, Houston, TX, USA

A major metabolic abnormality in diabetes mellitus (DM) is dyslipidemia, typically characterized by an elevation in serum triglyceride (TG) levels and a decrease in high-density lipoprotein cholesterol (HDL-C) levels. DM per se does not alter the serum low-density lipoprotein cholesterol (LDL-C) concentration, but for any given level of LDL-C, patients who are diabetic are more likely to suffer cardiovascular events than those who are not diabetic. Also, DM is often associated with elevated levels of non–HDL-C (Eq. 1) and typically has a preponderance of the more atherogenic smaller, denser low-density lipoprotein (LDL) particles, even when LDL-C levels are within the normal range [1], as demonstrated in the following equation:

$$\text{Non–HDL-C} = \text{TChol} - (\text{LDL-C} + \text{VLDL-C}) \quad (1)$$

where *TChol* is the amount of total cholesterol and *VLDL-C* is very low-density lipoprotein cholesterol.

Much of the excess mortality in type 2 diabetes (T2DM) is due to macrovascular complications (coronary artery, cerebrovascular, and peripheral vascular disease). Cardiovascular disease (CVD) accounts for approximately 70% of total mortality in T2DM; and all manifestations of CVD—namely, coronary artery disease (CAD), stroke, and peripheral vascular disease—are substantially more common (2–4 times)

in patients who have T2DM than in those who are not diabetic [2–5].

Pathophysiology of diabetic dyslipidemia

T2DM is associated with a cluster of interrelated plasma lipid and lipoprotein abnormalities, including reduced HDL-C, a predominance of small, dense LDL particles, and elevated TGs [6]. Similar changes are also seen in the metabolic syndrome, as defined by the National Cholesterol Education Program (NCEP) Adult Treatment Panel III (ATP III) (Box 1) [7,8]. The metabolic syndrome, discussed in detail elsewhere in this issue, is a constellation of risk factors whose presence predicts increased risk for both CVD and DM [8–10]. Insulin resistance has striking effects on lipoprotein size and on subclass particle concentrations, such as very low-density lipoprotein (VLDL), LDL, and high-density lipoprotein (HDL)] [11]. There is evidence that each of these dyslipidemic features is associated with increased risk of CVD. Several studies have established the association between LDL particle size or density and CAD [11–14].

Altered metabolism of TG-rich lipoproteins is an integral part of the atherogenic dyslipidemia seen in DM. Increased hepatic secretion of VLDL and decreased clearance of VLDL and intestinally derived chylomicrons result in prolonged plasma retention of these particles and accumulation of highly atherogenic, partially lipolyzed, cholesterol-enriched intermediate-density lipoprotein remnants (Fig. 1). Increased hepatic production and diminished plasma

* Corresponding author. Baylor College of Medicine Faculty Towers, 1709 Dryden Road, Suite 1000, Houston, TX 77030.
E-mail address: agarber@bcm.tmc.edu (A.J. Garber).

1551-7136/06/$ – see front matter © 2006 Elsevier Inc. All rights reserved.
doi:10.1016/j.hfc.2005.12.001

Box 1. Metabolic syndrome diagnosis needs 3 or more of the following National Cholesterol Education Program Adult Treatment Panel III criteria

1. Abdominal obesity
   (waist circumference)
   • Men > 102 cm (40 inches)
   • Women > 88 cm (35 inches)
2. Triglycerides ≥ 150 mg/dL
3. High-density lipoprotein
   (HDL) cholesterol
   • Men < 45 mg/dL
   • Women < 55 mg/dL
4. Blood pressure ≥ 135/85
5. Fasting glucose > 110 mg/dL[a]

[a] The new American Diabetes Association criterion for impaired fasting glucose is > 100 mg/dL [84].
Data from Expert Panel on Detection, Evaluation and Treatment of High Blood Cholesterol in Adults. Executive summary of the third report of the National Cholesterol Education Program (NCEP) Expert Panel on Detection, Evaluation, and Treatment of High Blood Cholesterol in Adults (Adult Treatment Panel III). JAMA 2001; 285:2486–97.

clearance of large VLDL result in increased production of precursors of small dense LDL particles [12–14].

Recent reports have indicated that LDL particle concentrations, and specifically levels of small dense LDL, are predictive of coronary events, independent of other coronary disease risk factors [13,14]. Seven distinct LDL subspecies differing in their metabolic behavior and pathological roles have been identified (Table 1). Plasma VLDL levels correlate with increased density and decreased size of LDL [15]. Small dense LDL particles appear to arise from the progressive intravascular processing of specific larger VLDL precursors through a series of steps, including lipolysis (see Fig. 1) [16]. Cholesterol ester transfer protein-mediated TG enrichment of lipolytic products and hepatic lipase-mediated hydrolysis of TG and phospholipids result in increased production of small dense LDL particles (see Fig. 1). The reduction in HDL-C seen in the metabolic syndrome and T2DM is

multifactorial, but an important factor is the increased transfer of cholesterol from HDL to TG-rich lipoproteins, with reciprocal transfer of TG to HDL. Hydrolysis of TG-rich HDL particles by hepatic lipase results in its rapid catabolism and clearance from plasma [17]. The usual pattern is one of low HDL_{2b}, and relative increases in the small dense subfractions HDL_{3b} and HDL_{3c}.

Lipotoxic heart disease

Early man went through cycles of food abundance and famine, and the evolution of the adipocyte perhaps enabled him to store excess energy substrate to sustain life through periods of starvation, especially since the tissues of the lean body mass lacked the ability to store triacylglycerols [18]. In contrast, modern existence, especially in the Western Hemisphere, is characterized by easy and affordable access to high-calorie food substrates and an increasingly sedentary lifestyle, resulting in a mismatch between energy consumption and expenditure. The result is an increasing incidence and prevalence of obesity, a state characterized by a pathological increase in subcutaneous, and more importantly, visceral fat mass. Hydrolysis of stored TGs releases free fatty acids (FFA). While FFA subserves important physiologic functions, chronically elevated plasma levels (such as those seen in obesity and T2DM) are deleterious, largely owing to the toxic effects in "lean" tissues. Even modest caloric surplus may lead to "ectopic" lipid deposition in liver, heart, muscle, and endocrine pancreas, resulting in nonalcoholic fatty liver disease, lipotoxic heart disease, and DM or insulin resistance. Excess presence of triacylglycerols beyond the oxidative needs of lean tissue (termed steatosis), leads to a FFA spillover effect, resulting in tissue dysfunction or lipotoxicity, largely caused by potentially toxic endproducts of nonoxidative FFA metabolism [19], eventually leading to lipoapoptosis or lipid-induced cell death (Fig. 2) [20]. The toxic consequences of lipid overload depend on the magnitude and duration of the imbalance between FFA influx and oxidation in any given tissue. In diet-induced obesity, for example, nonadipose tissue is protected by high leptin levels during the initial phase of FFA excess, but later leptin resistance of undetermined etiology sets in and seems to be responsible for gradual accrual of lipids in lean tissue, resulting in lipotoxicity [20]. Some of the mechanisms of lipotoxic damage, based on mouse data, are illustrated in Fig. 2. Hydrolysis of the TG stores results in expansion of the FFA pool, providing substrate for nonoxidative FFA metabolism. In a va-

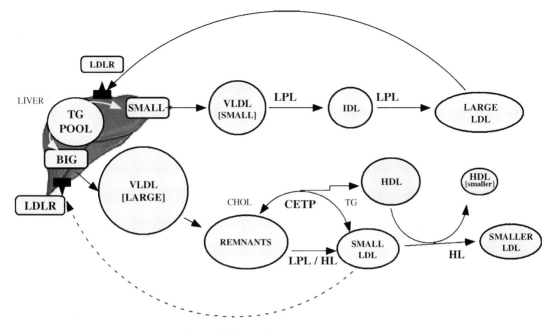

Low affinity pathway

Fig. 1. Altered triglyceride metabolism in diabetes mellitus leading to atherogenic lipoprotein phenotype. CETP, cholesterol ester transfer protein; HL, hepatic lipase; HDL, high-density lipoprotein; IDL, intermediate-density lipoprotein; LDL, low-density lipoprotein; LDLR, low density lipoprotein receptor; LPL, lipoprotein lipase, TG, triglyceride; VLDL, very low-density lipoprotein.

Table 1
Low-density lipoprotein and high-density lipoprotein subparticle changes in diabetic dyslipidemia

Lipoprotein subclass	Pattern seen in DM	Particle density (g/mL)
LDL_1	↓	1.019–1.023
LDL_{2a}	↓	1.023–1.028
LDL_{2b}	↓	1.028–1.034
LDL_{3a}	↑	1.034–1.041
LDL_{3b}	↑	1.041–1.044
LDL_{4a}	Variable	1.044–1.051
LDL_{4b}	Variable	1.051–1.063
HDL_{2b}	↓	1.063–1.100
HDL_{2a}	Variable	1.100–1.125
HDL_{3a}	Variable	1.125–1.147
HDL_{3b}	↑	1.147–1.167
HDL_{3c}	↑	1.167–1.200

Abbreviations: HDL, high-density lipoprotein; LDL, low-density lipoprotein; ↓, decreased; ↑, increased.
Data from Krauss RM. Lipids and lipoproteins in patients with type 2 diabetes. Diabetes Care 2004;27:1496–504.

riety of experimental systems [21–23], lipotoxicity from accumulation of long chain fatty acids seems related specifically to saturated fatty acids as opposed to unsaturated fatty acids. This selectivity has been attributed to the generation of specific proapoptotic lipid species or signaling molecules in response to saturated but not unsaturated fatty acids. The nature of such signals may differ across cell types, but includes reactive oxygen species generation [21], de novo ceramide synthesis [24], nitric oxide generation [25], decreases in phosphatidylinositol-3-kinase [26], and primary effects on mitochondrial structure or function [27]. Long chain fatty acids may also suppress antiapoptotic factors such as Bcl-2 [28]. Co-supplementation with monounsaturated fatty acids [26,29] has been shown to rescue saturated fatty-acid-induced lipoapoptosis by an unknown mechanism. In pancreatic cell [30] and in cardiac myocytes [31], the ceramide pathway seems to be most important of the harmful routes, although other mechanisms probably operate also.

The accumulation of TG in the heart, caused by a mismatch between the uptake and the oxidation of

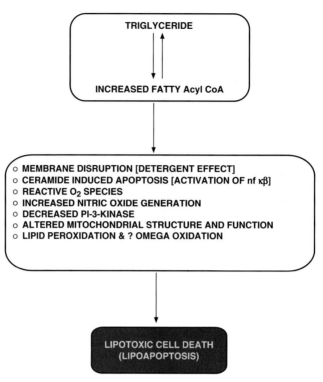

Fig. 2. Cellular mechanisms of lipotoxicity. NFκB, nuclear factor κB; O$_2$, oxygen.

fatty acids, has pathophysiologic implications. "Lipid cardiomyopathy" was identified more than 30 years ago in the hypertrophied hearts of mice rendered obese by the administration of gold thioglucose [32], and the deleterious effect of FFA on cardiac myocytes has been well-documented subsequently [22,33]. Patients who have congenital lipodystrophy, a rare disorder in which the absence of adipocytes results in the pathological accumulation of lipid of nonadipose (lean) tissues, and individuals who have inherited mitochondrial fatty acid oxidation defects develop premature cardiomyopathy [34,35]. In the Zucker diabetic fatty fa/fa rat, evidence of increased non-beta-oxidative fat acid metabolism in the myocardium is reflected by increases in myocardial TG and ceramide content [31] and by increased myocardial oxidative stress [36]. Myocardial expression of inducible nitric oxide synthase (iNOS) expression is high [31], and the increased nitric oxide is believed to interact with super oxide to induce apoptosis [37]. There is echocardiographic evidence of reduced myocardial contractility due to loss of functioning myocytes through apoptosis [31]. Excess FFAs themselves probably provide the signals for such metabolic adjustments by serving as ligands for

peroxisome proliferator-activating receptors (PPAR) [38]. These changes can be completely prevented by treatment with troglitazone, a PPARγ agonist that reduces the myocardial TG and ceramide content, preserves and promotes FFA re-esterification, and lowers FFA levels, thus leading to improved contractile function of the heart [31]. While PPARγ, a lipogenic transcription factor, is expressed at higher levels in adipose tissue, PPARα, a transcription factor that up-regulates several fatty acid oxidative enzymes, carnitine palmitoyl transferase-1 (CPT-1) and acyl CoA oxidase (ACO) [39,40], is expressed in lean tissues at relatively higher levels. It has been suggested that surplus fatty acids, in a compensated state, may up-regulate PPARα and the oxidative machinery, and thus prevent the overaccumulation of unoxidized lipids [41].

Dyslipidemia and cardiac dysfunction

While cardiac dysfunction in T2DM is multifactorial, dyslipidemia is a major contributory factor, especially with respect to CAD. Bell [42] coined the phrase "cardiotoxic triad" to refer to the simultaneous and deleterious presence of CAD, hypertension, and diabetic cardiomyopathy. While dyslipidemia has a prominent role in the genesis of CAD in the patient who is diabetic, its role in that of nonischemic diabetic heart disease and diabetic cardiomyopathy is less clear. At the level of the cardiac myocyte, several abnormalities have been described. DM results in a decrease in the volume fraction of myofibrils (F-actin) [43], sarcoplasmic reticulum, T-tubules, and cardiomyocyte diameter. Vacuoles and lipid droplets have also been observed in cardiac myocytes. Swelling of mitochondria occurs after a long spell of DM [44] and leads to the degeneration of the intra-axonal mitochondria. An abnormality of the cardiac interstitium, such as increased fibrosis, has been documented in patients who are normotensive and have type 1 DM [45]. Thickening of the basement membrane of the vessels of the heart has also been observed in a rat model of T2DM [46]. Remodeling of the extra cellular matrix proteins is a regular feature in DM, as is up-regulation of endothelin, a vasoactive substance that results in an increase in extra cellular matrix proteins, such as fibronectin and collagen type IV, and leads to the thickening of capillary endothelial basement membrane [47]. These changes, when coupled with the atherogenic lipoprotein profile seen in DM, result in small vessel occlusion and ischemia. Intracardiac neural changes have been described in diabetic animal models and in humans who are diabetic. Increased dysfunctional intra-axonal mitochondria, increased membrane fragments, and lamellar inclusion bodies are some of the changes seen within the myocardium in DM. In cardiac neuropathy, both the sensory and autonomic functions are impaired. Thus painless myocardial ischemia and reduced heart rate variability are common in patients who have long-term DM [48]. In part, the pathogenesis of cardiac neuropathy has been attributed to biochemical changes involving the accumulation of intracellular sorbitol, as excess glucose causes a shift in its metabolism by way of the polyol pathways [49]. Although the pathological basis of nonischemic diabetic cardiomyopathy has not been fully elucidated, involved mechanisms appear to include oxidative stress, formation of advanced glycation products, and abnormal intracellular calcium handling by the cardiac myocytes.

Heart failure: the final scourge

Clinical cardiac dysfunction in the patient who is diabetic may manifest in one of three ways: CAD/ischemic cardiomyopathy, "diabetic" (nonischemic) cardiomyopathy, or autonomic dysfunction of the heart. Any combination of these may occur, resulting in a gradual loss of functioning cardiac myocytes, which results in decompensated heart disease and the syndrome of congestive heart failure. Framingham data suggests that the relative risk for congestive heart failure for men and women who are diabetic is approximately twofold and fivefold greater, respectively, than that of the general population [5]. The Acute Decompensated Heart Failure National Registry (ADHERE) revealed that approximately 44% of patients hospitalized with acutely decompensated heart failure have DM [50]. In the Western Hemisphere, congestive heart failure is closely related to CAD; however, there has been an increase in the prevalence of heart failure despite a decline in CAD-related mortality [51]. Increased predilection to heart failure in DM may be due to several factors. First, DM is a risk factor for the development of coronary atherosclerosis and its complications, such as myocardial infarction [52], with critical loss of functioning myocardium. Second, hypertension, a factor pathophysiologically linked to 70% of all congestive heart failure cases, frequently coexists with DM [52,53]. Third, "diabetic" cardiomyopathy, initially described by Rubler and colleagues [54], and discussed in greater detail elsewhere in this issue, contributes to additional increased risk of heart failure in these patients [55]. In a large diabetes-registry-based cohort study [56], after adjustment for several factors, including age, sex, ethnicity, cigarette smoking, hypertension, obesity, type and duration of diabetes, and incidence of interim myocardial infarction, each 1% increase in hemoglobin (Hb) A_{1c} was associated with an 8% increased risk of heart failure (95% CI 5–12). An Hb A_{1c} greater than or equal to 10, relative to Hb A_{1c} less than 7, was associated with 1.56-fold (95% CI 1.26–1.93) greater risk of heart failure. In the United Kingdom Prospective Diabetes Study (UKPDS) [57], each 1% increase in Hb A_{1C} conferred a 12% increase in the risk of heart failure. There was a linear relationship between increasing Hb A_{1c} concentration and the incidence of heart failure cases (Table 2) [57]. The prevalence of diabetes is even higher in registries of patients hospitalized with heart failure, ranging from 26% to 44% [58].

Lessons learned from randomized controlled clinical trials on the management of diabetic dyslipidemia

The Executive Summary of the Third Report of the National Cholesterol Education Program Expert

Table 2
Incidence of heart failure in patients who have type 2 diabetes mellitus by category of updated mean hemoglobin A_{1c} concentration in percent

Criteria	Mean HbA_{1c} concentration (%)					
	<6	6−7	7−8	8−9	9−10	10−11
Events/person years	17/9967	34/12928	36/9782	20/6432	10/3062	10/1514
Unadjusted rate[a]	1.7	2.6	3.7	3.1	3.3	6.6
Adjusted rate[b]	2.3	3.4	5.0	4.4	5.0	11.9
(95% CI)	(1.2−4.5)	(1.9 to 5.8)	(2.9 to 8.6)	(2.4 to 8.2)	(2.3 to 10.6)	(5.5 to 25.8)

[a] Person years, events, and unadjusted rates are for all patients.

[b] Rates per 1000 person years' follow-up adjusted in Poisson regression model to white men aged 50−54 y at diagnosis of diabetes and followed up for 7.5 to <12.5 y, termed "10 years" (n = 4585).
Data from Stratton IM, Adler AI, Neil HA, et al. Association of glycaemia with macrovascular and microvascular complications of type 2 diabetes (UKPDS 35): prospective observational study. BMJ 2000;321:405−12.

Panel on Detection, Evaluation, and Treatment of High Blood Cholesterol in Adults (ATP III) was published in May 2001 [7] and updated in 2004 [8]. The update followed publication of results from several large trials of statin therapy with observed clinical endpoints.

Several primary and secondary prevention trials have reported diabetes-specific outcomes in their reports (Table 3). Of note, the Heart Protection Study [59] randomized 5963 patients aged greater than 40 years who had diabetes and total cholesterol greater than 135 mg/dL. In this trial, patients assigned

Table 3
Effectiveness of lipid-lowering therapy in diabetes mellitus: subgroup analyses from various primary and secondary prevention trials

Study, year [Ref.]	CHD event rate (n/N)		RR (95% CI) for CHD event	ARR in CHD events	NNT
	Controls	Intervention group			
Primary prevention trials					
AFCAPS/TexCAPS, 1998 [86]	6/71	4/84	0.56 (0.17−1.92)	0.040	27.1
ALLHAT-LLT, 2002 [63]	NR	NR	0.89 (0.71−1.10)	NR	NR
ASCOT-LLA, 2003 [87]	46/1274	38/1258	0.84 (0.55−1.29)	0.010	169.5
CARDS, 2004 [60]	129/1410	83/1428	0.63 (0.48−0.83)	0.032	31.3
HHS, 1992 [88]	8/76	2/59	0.32 (0.07−1.46)	0.070	14.0
HPS, 2002 [89]	367/1976	276/2006	0.74 (0.64−0.85)	0.050	20.8
PROSPER, 2002 [90]	28/205	32/209	1.23 (0.77−1.95)	−0.030	−32.3
Secondary prevention trials					
4S, 1997 [91]	44/97	24/105	0.50 (0.33−0.76)	0.230	4.4
CARE, 1996 [92]	112/304	81/282	0.78 (0.62−0.99)	0.080	12.3
HPS, 2004 [85]	381/1009	325/972	0.89 (0.79−1.00)	0.040	23.1
LIPID, 1998 [93]	88/386	76/396	0.84 (0.64−1.11)	0.040	27.7
LIPS, 2002 [94]	31/82	26/120	0.53 (0.29−0.97)	0.160	6.2
POST-CABG, 1999 [95]	14/53	9/63	0.53 (0.18−1.60)	0.120 (0.030−0.270)	8.2
PROSPER, 2002 [90]	31/115	38/112	1.26 (0.85−1.87)	−0.070 (0.190−0.050)	−14.3
VA-HIT, 1999 [96,97]	116/318	88/309	0.76 (0.57−1.01)	0.080 (0.010−0.150)	12.5

Abbreviations: AFCAPS/TexCAPS, Air Force Coronary Atherosclerosis Prevention Study/Texas Coronary Atherosclerosis Prevention Study; ALLHAT-LLT, Antihypertensive and Lipid-Lowering Treatment to Prevent Heart Attack Trial–Lipid-Lowering Trial; ARR, absolute risk reduction; ASCOT-LLA, Anglo-Scandinavian Cardiac Outcomes Trial–Lipid-Lowering Arm; CARDS, Collaborative atorvastatin diabetes study; CARE, Cholesterol and Recurrent Events trial; CHD, coronary heart disease; CI, confidence interval; HHS, Helsinki Heart Study; HPS, Heart Protection Study; LIPID, Long-Term Intervention with Pravastatin in Ischemic Disease trial; LIPS, Lescol Intervention Prevention Study; NNT, number needed to treat; NR, not reported; Post-CABG, Post−Coronary Artery Bypass Graft trial; PROSPER, Prospective Study of Pravastatin in the Elderly at Risk; RR, relative risk; 4S, Scandinavian Simvastatin Survival Study; VA-HIT, Veterans Administration High-Density Lipoprotein Cholesterol Intervention Trial.

to simvastatin had a 22% reduction (95% CI 13–30) in the event rate for major CVD events. This risk reduction was similar across all LDL subcategories examined, including patients who had lower pretreatment LDL cholesterol levels (< 116 mg/dL) and those who did not have identified vascular disease [59]. The Collaborative Atorvastatin Diabetes Study (CARDS) multicenter study [60] was a primary prevention trial that randomized 2838 patients aged 40 to 75 years who had diabetes to placebo (n = 1410; mean baseline LDL-C 118 mg/dl) or atorvastatin, 10 mg/d (n = 1428; mean baseline LDL-C 119 mg/dl). Eighty percent of the atorvastatin-treated group and 25% of the placebo group achieved their target plasma level of LDL-C (100 mg/dL). At the end of the trial (just under 5 years), there was a 37% relative risk reduction in cardiovascular events associated with the atorvastatin group. In favor of aggressive statin therapy are the results of the Pravastatin or Atorvastatin Evaluation and Infection Therapy (PROVE-IT) study [61], which randomized 4162 patients who had acute coronary syndrome to receive either atorvastatin, 80 mg/d (n = 2099; 17.5% who had T2DM), or pravastatin, 40 mg/d (n = 2063; 17.8% who had T2DM), for an average of 1.5 years. Patients randomized to atorvastatin, 80 mg/d, had a 16% lower risk of a CVD composite endpoint (P < .01); and cardiovascular benefit from aggressive LDL-C lowering was seen in patients who had T2DM and those who did not. In the Treat to New Targets (TNT) study [62], a secondary prevention study, 10,003 men and women aged 35 to 75 years were randomized to receive atorvastatin, 10 mg/d (n = 5006) or 80 mg/d (n = 4995), and followed for an average 5-year period. Fifteen percent in each treatment arm had T2DM. Overall analysis showed a primary event rate of 10.9% and 8.7% in the low- and high-dose atorvastatin groups, respectively. This outcome represented a 2.2% absolute risk reduction and 22% relative risk reduction. A meta-analysis [62] evaluated the effectiveness of lipid lowering drug therapy on outcomes in patients who had T2DM, including data from six primary prevention and eight secondary prevention trials (Table 4; meta-analysis did not

Table 4
An overview of lipid-lowering agents

Drug	Major indication	Daily dosage range	Mechanism
Statins			
Atorvastatin	↑ LDL-C	10–80 mg	↓ Cholesterol synthesis
Fluvastatin	↑ LDL-C	20–80 mg	↑ LDL-C clearance (receptor mediated)
Lovastatin	↑ LDL-C	20–80 mg	
Pravastatin	↑ LDL-C	40–80 mg	
Rosuvastatin	↑ LDL-C	10–40 mg	
Simvastatin	↑ LDL-C	20–80 mg	
BAS			
Cholestyramine	↑ LDL-C	4–32 g	↑ Bile acid excretion
Colestipol	↑ LDL-C	5–40 g	↑ LDL-C clearance (receptor mediated)
Colesevelam	↑ LDL-C	3.75–4.375 g	
Niacin			
Immediate-release	↑ TG and LDL-C ↓HDL-C	100 mg–2 g tid	↓ Hepatic VLDL synthesis ↓ Lp(a)
Sustained-release	↑ TG and LDL-C ↓HDL-C	250 mg–1.5 g bid	
Extended-release	↑ TG and LDL-C ↓ HDL-C	500 mg–2 g qhs	
Fibrates			
Gemfibrozil	↑ TG and Lp remnants	600 mg qod–600 mg bid	↑ LPL activity ↓ apo C-III synthesis and VLDL production
Fenofibrate	↑ TG and Lp remnants	54 mg qod–160 mg bid	
Fish oils	↑ TG	3–12 g[a]	↓ VLDL production
CAI			
Ezetimibe	↑ LDL-C	10 mg/d	↓ cholesterol absorption ↑ LDL-C clearance

Abbreviations: apo, apolipoprotein; BAS, bile acid sequestrants; bid, twice a day; CAI, cholesterol absorption inhibitor; g, grams; HDL-C, high-density lipoprotein cholesterol; Lp, lipoprotein; LPL, lipoprotein lipase; qhs, every night; qod, once a day; TG, triglyceride; tid, three times a day; ↓, decreased; ↑, increased.

[a] Dose refers to total content of eicosa pentanoic acid (EPA) + docosa hexanoic acid (DHA).

include data from CARDS trial [60]). For primary prevention, over a weighted trial average of 4.3 years, the pooled relative risk for cardiovascular events with lipid-lowering therapy was 0.78 (95% CI 0.67–0.89), absolute risk reduction was 0.03 (95% less CI 0.01–0.04), and the estimate of the number needed to treat to prevent an event was 34.5. The investigators included results of the Antihypertensive and Lipid-Lowering Treatment to Prevent Heart Attack Trial (ALLHAT) (see Table 4) [63] in the pooled estimates of relative risk but not those of absolute risk reduction because these data were not available. For secondary prevention, over a weighted trial average of 4.9 years, the pooled relative risk for cardiovascular events was similar to that for primary prevention, at 0.76 (95% CI 0.59–0.93); but because of the greater absolute risk of those who had known coronary artery disease, the pooled absolute risk reduction was more than twice as high, at 0.07 (95% CI 0.03–0.12), and the number needed to treat for benefit was only 13.8. As in the Heart Protection Study [59], the statin was equally effective in individuals who had high and low levels of plasma LDL-C. In CARDS [60], atorvastatin significantly reduced the incidence of both stroke and CAD.

In November 2005, the results of the Fenofibrate Intervention and Event Lowering in Diabetes (FIELD) trial were presented in the American Heart Association annual meeting and simultaneously published early online by *The Lancet* [64]. This study randomized 9795 diabetic individuals who had T2DM to either micronized fenofibrate (n = 4895) or placebo (n = 4900) and followed them for a period of 5 years. Fenofibrate was associated with a nonsignificant reduction in the primary endpoint, a composite of nonfatal myocardial infarction or coronary heart disease (CHD) death (5.9% versus 5.2%, placebo versus active treatment: hazard ratio = 0.89). Fibrate therapy reduced nonfatal myocardial infarction by 24% (P = .010), but this result was offset by a 19% increase in CHD death (P = .22) versus placebo. In terms of secondary endpoints, fibrate therapy was associated with a significant reduction in total cardiovascular events (CVD death, myocardial infarction, stroke, and coronary and carotid revascularization). The relative risk was 11% lower with fenofibrate versus placebo (P = .035), with the benefit being driven primarily by a reduction in coronary revascularizations and nonfatal myocardial infarctions. Subgroup analysis revealed that the beneficial effect of fibrates on total cardiovascular events was greatest in patients free of CVD at baseline, in which the hazard ratio was 0.85 versus placebo. Fibrates also appeared to be more effective in patients aged

less than 65 years than in older patients, but the numbers were too small to draw firm conclusions. Otherwise, the benefits were similar irrespective of gender, HDL cholesterol, TGs, and presence of dyslipidemia at baseline. Tertiary analyses showed that fibrates were significantly superior to placebo with respect to progression of microalbuminuria, need for retinal laser therapy, hospitalizations for angina pectoris, and amputations. Active therapy, however, was also associated with significantly more cases of pulmonary embolism and pancreatitis than placebo. The observed effects of fenofibrate in this study were affected by differential statin use, because patients in the placebo group were more than twice as likely as those treated with fenofibrate to be started on a statin during the study, with an identical dropout rate. The FIELD study results do not preclude use of fibrates in the context of established statin therapy in those who have DM; and its main use will likely continue to be as part of a combination lipid drug regimen, because the drug is usually well-tolerated alone and in combination with statins.

Clinical trial data on the use of niacin in the patient who has diabetes

Concern has been raised about the adverse glycemic effects of nicotinic acid (niacin) in patients who are diabetic. Using a randomized crossover design, Garg and Grundy [65] studied the efficacy of niacin monotherapy in patients who had diabetic dyslipidemia. Compared with the control period, nicotinic acid therapy reduced the plasma TChol level by 24%, TG by 45%, VLDL-C by 58%, and LDL-C by 15%, and increased HDL-C by 34%. However, niacin therapy resulted in a 16% increase in mean plasma glucose concentrations and a 21% increase in Hb A_{1c}.

The Assessment of Diabetes Control and Evaluation of the efficacy of Niaspan Trial (ADVENT) [66] assessed the efficacy, safety, and tolerability of once-daily extended-release niacin in the treatment of dyslipidemia associated with T2DM. During a 16-week, double-blind, placebo-controlled trial, 148 patients were randomized to placebo (n = 49) or 1000 mg/d (n = 45) or 1500 mg/d (n = 52) of extended-release niacin. Sixty-nine patients (47%) were also receiving concomitant therapy with statins. Dose-dependent increases in HDL-C levels (+19% to +24%, P < .05) versus placebo for both niacin dosages) and reductions in TG levels (−13% to −28%, P < .05) versus placebo for the 1500-mg extended-release niacin) were observed. Baseline and week 16 values for HbA_{1c} were 7.13% and 7.11%, respectively, in the placebo group; 7.28% and 7.35%, respectively, in the 1000-mg extended-release niacin group ($P = .16$ versus placebo); and 7.2% and 7.5% respectively in the 1500-mg extended-release niacin group ($P = .048$ versus placebo). Only four patients discontinued participation because of altered glucose control. Rates of adverse events other than flushing were similar for the niacin and placebo groups. Four patients discontinued participation because of flushing (including one receiving placebo). No hepatotoxicity effects or myopathy were observed.

In another study [67], niacin at lower doses (1000 mg/d) in combination with a pravastatin (20 mg/d) was more effective than pravastatin (40 mg/d) alone in lowering serum TG and elevating HDL-C. The combination was more effective than niacin (1500 mg/d) alone in reducing TChol, TG, and LDL-C levels. In this study, combination therapy proved equally effective in individuals who had and who did not have T2DM.

The Arterial Disease Multiple Intervention Trial (ADMIT) [68] randomized 468 patients who had peripheral arterial disease, including 125 who had T2DM, to receive niacin (crystalline nicotinic acid), 3000 mg/d or maximum tolerated dosage (n = 64 who had diabetes; n = 173 who did not have diabetes), or placebo (n = 61 who had diabetes; n = 170 who did not have diabetes) for up to 60 weeks (12-week active run-in and 48-week double-blind). In participants who had and did not have diabetes, niacin use significantly increased HDL-C by 29% and 29%, decreased TGs by 23% and 28%, and decreased LDL-C by 8% and 9%, respectively, ($P < .001$ for niacin versus placebo for all). Glucose levels were modestly increased by niacin, 8.7 mg/dL and 6.3 mg/dL (0.4 mmol/L and 0.3 mmol/L, $P = .04$ and $P < .001$), in participants who had and who did not have diabetes, respectively; but Hb A_{1c} levels were unchanged from baseline to follow-up in participants who had diabetes treated with niacin.

Treatment considerations in diabetic dyslipidemia

At present, the American Diabetes Association (ADA) [69] and the NCEP [8] recommend that normalization of elevated plasma LDL-C is the first priority in treating diabetic dyslipidemia. The choice of secondary and tertiary targets, however, differs slightly between the NCEP and the ADA. The NCEP recommends that after the primary target for LDL-C is reached, if the plasma TG level is greater than 200 mg/dL (2.26 mmol/L), then non-HDL should be considered as a secondary target. The non-HDL cholesterol goal is set 30 mg/dL above the LDL-C goal; and thus for diabetics, it is set at less than or equal to 130 mg/dL (3.37 mmol/L). The ADA secondary and tertiary targets are to raise plasma HDL-C and lower plasma TG levels, respectively. The ADA and the NCEP have the same LDL-C goal of less than or equal to 100 mg/dL (2.59 mmol/L). The 2005 ADA recommendations [70] suggest that health care providers should aim for an LDL reduction of 30% to 40%. In tandem, the latest NCEP update [8] suggests a reduction by 40%. Both the ADA [69] and the NCEP [8] recommend treatment of dyslipidemia in patients who have diabetes to the same degree of intensity as that for patients who have CAD (eg, treat diabetes as a CAD risk equivalent). This designation was based on evidence that most patients who have diabetes have a relatively high 10-year risk for developing CVD. Haffner and colleagues [4] showed that over a 7 year period, diabetic patients who do not have prior myocardial infarction have as high a risk of myocardial infarction as nondiabetic patients who have previous myocardial infarction. In addition, the onset of CVD in patients who have diabetes carries a poor prognosis, both at the time of an acute CVD event and in the postevent period.

Patients who have both DM and CVD are at very high risk for future CVD events, as was shown by the Heart Protection Study [59]. In terms of absolute risk reduction, this category of patients obtained the greatest benefit from statin therapy. The Heart Protection Study included several different types of high-risk patients that would qualify as CHD risk equivalents according to ATP III. The benefit of LDL-lowering therapy in such high-risk patients was amply demonstrated by the Heart Protection Study. Therefore, patients who have the combination of DM and CVD deserve intensive lipid-lowering therapy; and it is reasonable to attempt to achieve a very low LDL-C level (< 70 mg/dL) in this group. On the other hand, in those who have DM without CVD, with baseline LDL-C less than or equal to 116 mg/dL, risk reduction accompanying statin therapy was only marginally significant for first coronary event. Thus, in this group, the option to start an LDL-lowering drug when LDL-C is less than 100 mg/dL must be determined based on the overall CVD risk estimate of the patient in question. The ATP III panel [8] pointed out that some diabetic patients may not have a CHD risk equivalent. For example, for younger diabetics who do not have other CVD risk factors, an LDL-C level less than 130 mg/dL might be a more appropriate cutoff point for pharmacotherapy. The investigators also proposed that a minimal "standard" statin dose be chosen if CVD prevention is to be successful, meaning at least 30%–40% decrease in LDL-C.

Several studies have looked at the predictive efficacy of non–HDL-C (composed of all atherogenic lipoprotein subfractions, namely, VLDL, intermediate-density lipoprotein, and LDL} in predicting cardiovascular endpoints in individuals who are diabetic. In the Health Professionals' Follow-up Study [71], non–HDL-C was a strong predictor of CVD in 746 diabetic men aged 46 to 81 years during a 6-year follow-up. In a Finnish study [72], 1059 middle-aged men and women who had T2DM were followed for 7 years; and it was found that higher levels of non–HDL-C were independently associated with a twofold increase in the risk for CHD death or morbidity. In the Strong Heart Study cohort [73] of 2108 American-Indian men and women aged 45 to 74 years who had diabetes, the hazard ratios for the highest tertile of non–HDL-C were higher than those for LDL-C among diabetic men and women. A more recent prospective cohort study [74] pooled data from four publicly available data sets, confining eligible subjects to white individuals aged greater than 30 years and free of CHD at baseline (12,660 men and 6721 women). Diabetes status was defined as either "reported by physician—diagnosed and on medication" or having a fasting glucose level greater than or equal to 126 mg/dL at the baseline examination. The primary endpoint was CHD death. Multivariate analysis of the pooled data showed that CHD risk in those who had DM did not increase with increasing LDL-C, but did increase with increasing non–HDL-C, suggesting that the latter is a stronger predictor of CHD death.

Based on current data, the following general recommendations can be made regarding diabetic dyslipidemia:

(1) LDL-C lowering is first priority. Once this lowering is accomplished, therapy to increase HDL-C and lower TG (non–LDL-C) must be initiated. A non–HDL-C level of greater than 130 mg% is a marker of increased cardiovascular morbidity and mortality in patients who are diabetic.
2. Statins should be used for primary prevention against macrovascular complications in patients (both men and women) who have T2DM and other cardiovascular risk factors.
3. Lipid-lowering therapy for secondary prevention must be offered to all individuals (men and women) who have diabetes and CHD.

4. Those eligible for statin treatment should at least receive moderate doses of the statin from the time of instituting the drug therapy.

More specific treatment guidelines for diabetic dyslipidemia are summarized in Box 2. Therapeutic

---

Box 2. Diabetic dyslipidemia: treatment goals

1. LDL-C
   - LDL-C goal < 100 mb/dL; < 70 mg/dL for very high-risk subjects (eg, those who have CVD)
   - LDL-C ≥;100 mg/dL; drug therapy beneficial in patients who have a CHD risk equivalent
   - LDL-C ≥130 mg/dL; pharmacotherapy recommended in all subjects
2. Triglyceride/non–HDL-C
   - Triglyceride 150–199 mg/dL; emphasis on weight reduction and physical activity
   - Triglyceride > 200 mg/dL; non–HDL-C goal < 130 mg/dL
   - Non–HDL-C > 130 mg/dL; consider drug therapy
3. HDL-C
   - Low HDL-C < 40 mg/dL; no goals for increasing HDL-C
   - Isolated low HDL-C (triglyceride < 200 mg/dL); fibrates or niacin can be considered

Data from Expert Panel on Detection, Evaluation and Treatment of High Blood Cholesterol in Adults. Executive summary of the third report of the National Cholesterol Education Program (NCEP) Expert Panel on Detection, Evaluation, and Treatment of High Blood Cholesterol in Adults (Adult Treatment Panel III). JAMA 2001; 285:2486–97; and Grundy SM, Cleeman JI, Merz CN, et al; for the Coordinating Committee of the National Cholesterol Education Program. Grundy SM, et al. Implications of recent clinical trials for the National Cholesterol Education Program Adult Treatment Panel III guidelines. J Am Coll Cardiol 2004;44:720–32.

lifestyle modification (exercise and diet therapy) are appropriate first measures for all patients who have diabetic dyslipidemia. Tight glycemic control and aggressive management of coexisting conditions such as obesity, hypertension, and other risk factors according to prescribed standards [70] are important in reducing morbidity and mortality in all patients who are diabetic. A detailed discussion on the various drugs and their safety profiles is beyond the scope of this review, but a summary of available lipid-lowering drugs appears in Table 4. LDL-C lowering is achieved mainly with statins. Fibrates effectively lower TG levels and raise HDL-C levels. Omega-3 fatty acids (fish oils) have an established role as an adjunct agent in lowering TG. Niacin preparations lower LDL-C and TG levels, and are the most effective drugs currently available for increasing HDL-C and lowering lipoprotein (a).

The complementary lipid-altering effects of statins and fibric acid derivatives (fibrates) have led to an increasing use of statin/fibrate combination therapy, particularly for patients who have the metabolic syndrome and DM, where the prevalence of mixed dyslipidemia is common. A recent retrospective analysis by Jones and Davidson [75] looking at the muscle effects, including rhabdomyolysis, in those on a statin-fibrate combination, as reported in the US Food and Drug Administration's Adverse Event Reporting System, found that fenofibrate resulted in a 15 times lower rhabdomyolysis reporting rate than did gemfibrozil, suggesting that it may be safer to use fenofibrate than gemfibrozil with a statin. Table 5 summarizes combination lipid therapy strategies.

Scant data exist on lipid-lowering therapy in patients who have type 1 DM. In the Heart Protection Study [59], approximately 600 patients who had type1 DM had a proportionately similar, but statistically insignificant risk reduction as in those who had T2DM. Although conclusive clinical trial data support is lacking, consideration ought to be given to

similar lipid-lowering therapy in patients who have type 1 DM as in T2DM (particularly if they have other cardiovascular risk factors or features of the metabolic syndrome), until data from clinical trials with sufficient power to look at clinical endpoints in those who have type 1 DM are available.

Antidiabetic therapy and lipids

By improving the diabetic-state insulin resistance, antidiabetic agents may influence lipid levels in individuals who have DM and dyslipidemia. In addition, they may have effects on the serum lipid profile, independent of their hypoglycemic effects. Controlled clinical trials suggest that metformin may contribute to lowering LDL-C and TG levels [76,77]. The thiazolidinedione group of agents (rosiglitazone and pioglitazone) may have certain lipid benefits. HDL-C levels may increase and TG concentrations frequently fall with thiazolidinedione therapy [78,79]. The effect on LDL-C is more variable, with increases reported with some [79,80] but not all [78] studies. In July 2005, the GLAI multicentric study [81] results suggested greater lipid effects of pioglitazone as compared with rosiglitazone. The potential beneficial effects of pioglitazone were not corroborated by the PROspective Pioglitazone Clinical Trial in Macrovascular Events (PROactive) study [82], however. This study was a prospective, randomized controlled trial in 5238 patients who had T2DM (mean follow-up of 34.5 months) with evidence of macrovascular disease, comparing pioglitazone (titrated from 15 mg–45 mg; n = 2605) or placebo (n = 2633), to be taken in addition to their glucose-lowering drugs and other medications. The primary composite endpoint was reduced by 10%, but did not reach statistical significance ($P = .095$). The so-called "secondary composite endpoint" of life-threatening events showed that pioglitazone significantly reduced the combined, but not the individual, risk of nonfatal heart attacks, strokes, and deaths, by 16% ($P = .027$). HDL-C increased (+19.0% pioglitazone versus +10.1% placebo, $P < .001$) and TG levels decreased (−11.4% pioglitazone versus +1.8% placebo, $P < .001$). LDL-C increased in both arms, albeit more in the pioglitazone group ($P \leq .003$).

The Simvastatin Thiazolidinedione Study Group [83] trial was a multicenter, randomized, double-blind, placebo-controlled trial that assessed the efficacy and tolerability of adding simvastatin, 40 mg, to existing thiazolidinedione therapy in patients who had T2DM (Hb $A_{1c} < 9\%$; LDL-C > 100 mg/dl). The primary endpoint was lowering LDL-C concen-

Table 5
Combination lipid therapy choices

Lipid abnormality	Suggested combination
Elevated LDL-C and TG <200 mg/dL	Statin + resin[a] or ezetimibe Statin + niacin + resin[a] or ezetimibe
Elevated LDL-C and TG 200–500 mg/dL and non–HDL-C >200 mg/dL	Statin + fibrate or niacin ± ω-3 fatty acids Resin[a] or ezetimibe + niacin or fibrate
Elevated TG >500 mg/dL	Niacin + fibrate ± ω-3 fatty acids

[a] Refers to bile acid sequestrants.

trations. The 253 patients (127 men, 126 women; mean age, 56 years) were randomized to either simvastatin or placebo (123 and 130 respectively). After 24 weeks, mean LDL-C concentrations were reduced 34% from baseline in the simvastatin group and were unchanged in the placebo group ($P < .001$). Compared with placebo, simvastatin produced significant reductions in concentrations of TChol, TG, non–HDL-C, and apolipoprotein (apo) B (all, $P < .001$) and significant increases in concentrations of HDL-C ($P = .002$) and apo A-I ($P = .006$). In patients who had not attained target concentrations of LDL-C (<100 mg/dL), TG (<150 mg/dL), or HDL-C (>45 mg/dL) at baseline, significantly more simvastatin recipients had achieved these goals at the end of the study compared with placebo recipients (LDL-C 67.3% versus 5.2%, $P < .001$; HDL-C 95.3% versus 83.6%, $P < .05$; and TG 40.8% versus 11.0%, $P < .001$, respectively).

It must be borne in mind that in those who have hyperglycemia, extreme insulin resistance, and deteriorating beta cell function, initiating insulin therapy, besides improving glucose control, may have a beneficial effect in lowering serum TG and potentially raising HDL-C levels. However, very high serum TG levels (>500 mg/dL) in an individual who is diabetic, especially when the glycemic control is satisfactory as evidenced by near-normal Hb A_{1c} levels, may suggest the copresence of a genetic hyperlipidemia, such as lipoprotein lipase or apo C-II deficiency, resulting in elevations in chylomicrons and /or VLDL (types 1 and V hyperlipoproteinemia), dysbetalipoproteinemia (type III hyperlipoproteinemia), or autosomal dominant familial hypertriglyceridemia. In addition to optimal oral hypoglycemic agent (OHA)/insulin therapy, therapy for these disorders will likely need specific TG-lowering agents, such as a fibrate or niacin or a combination of both, to lower TG levels to less than 500 mg/dL and minimize the risk of pancreatitis, a potentially life-threatening complication.

Diabetes, lipids, and cardiovascular endpoints – ongoing clinical trials

Several trials currently underway will address various issues regarding cardiovascular endpoints in individuals who are diabetic. The Look AHEAD (Action for Health in Diabetes) [84] trial will follow 5000 obese patients (55–75 years of age) who have T2DM for up to 11.5 years and will compare the effects of two interventions, lifestyle intervention or diabetes support and education, on major cardiovascular events. The NHLBI-led Action to Control Cardiovascular Risk in Diabetes (ACCORD) trial [85] is designed to test the effects on major CVD events of (1) intensive glycemia control (HbA$_{1C}$ target <6.0% versus 7.0–7.9%); (2) fibrate treatment to increase HDL-C and lower TG (in the context of good LDL-C and glycemic control); and (3) intensive blood pressure control (systolic blood pressure target of < 120 mm Hg versus < 140 mm Hg in the context of good glycemic control). All 10,000 middle-aged or older participants who have T2DM will be in the glycemia trial. In addition, one 2 × 2 trial will also address the lipid question in 5800 of the participants; and the other 2 × 2 trial will address the blood pressure question in 4200 of the participants. The Atorvastatin Study for Prevention of Coronary Heart Disease Endpoints in Non Insulin Dependent Diabetes Mellitus (ASPEN, n = 2421) [85] will randomize 2421 subjects who have T2DM with or without a previous myocardial infarction, to either atorvastatin, 10 mg, or placebo with cardiovascular endpoints similar to that of the CARDS trial [60], discussed previously. This trial will have at least 4 years of follow-up.

Summary

Current evidence supports the idea that all patients who have DM be treated to the same lipid goals, as are patients who have CAD. The first priority for treating dyslipidemia in T2DM is to lower plasma levels of LDL-C. The use of statins should be nearly universal in this population. The current literature lends support for empirical use of at least moderate doses of statins than it does for targeting specific LDL-C levels. There is a consensus that a minimal goal should be a plasma level of LDL-C of < 100 mg/dL (< 2.59 mmol/L). Although definitive data is lacking, an LDL-C goal of < 70 mg/dL (< 1.81 mmol/L) may be appropriate in some patients who have T2DM who are at very high risk, such as those who have prevalent CVD. Combination therapy may be indicated in many patients who have diabetes to achieve target LDL-C and non–LDL-C goals. When a statin–fibrate combination therapy is used, fenofibrate may be preferable to gemfibrozil. Ensuring good glycemic control and treating comorbid conditions, such as hypertension and obesity, according to established guidelines using a comprehensive, multidisciplinary approach, is key to diminishing morbidity and lowering mortality in individuals who have DM. The presumed lipid benefits of any specific antidiabetic agent must not be the primary reason for choosing that agent in a given patient. Such considerations are of secondary importance and merely play an adjunctive role in the lipid management of individuals who are diabetic. In most people who have diabetic dyslipidemia, specific lipid-lowering drugs, either alone or in combination, will be required to achieve LDL-C and non–HDL-C goals.

References

[1] Krauss RM. Lipids and lipoproteins in patients with type 2 diabetes. Diabetes Care 2004;27:1496–504.

[2] Pyorala K, Laakso M, Uusitupa M. Diabetes and atherosclerosis: an epidemiologic view. Diabetes Metabolism Reviews 1987;3:463–524.

[3] Laakso M, Lehto S. Epidemiology of risk factors for cardiovascular disease in diabetes and impaired glucose tolerance. Atherosclerosis 1998;137(Suppl): S65–73.

[4] Haffner SM, Lehto S, Ronnemaa T, et al. Mortality from coronary heart disease in subjects with type 2 diabetes and in non-diabetic subjects with and without prior myocardial infarction. N Engl J Med 1998;339:229–34.

[5] Kannel WB, McGee DL. Diabetes and cardiovascular disease. The Framingham study. JAMA 1979; 11(241):2035–8.

[6] Haffner SM. Management of dyslipidemia in adults with diabetes. Diabetes Care 2003;26(Suppl 1):S83–6.

[7] Expert Panel on Detection. Evaluation and treatment of high blood cholesterol in adults: Executive Summary of the Third report of the National Cholesterol Education Program (NCEP) expert panel on detection, evaluation, and treatment of high blood cholesterol in adults (adult treatment panel III). JAMA 2001;285:2486–97.

[8] Grundy SM, Cleeman JI, Merz CN, et al. Implications of recent clinical trials for the National Cholesterol Education Program adult treatment panel III guidelines. J Am Coll Cardiol 2004;44:720–32.

[9] Haffner SM, Mykkanen L, Festa A, et al. Insulin-resistant prediabetic subjects have more atherogenic risk factors than insulin-sensitive prediabetic subjects: implications for preventing coronary heart disease during the prediabetic state. Circulation 2000;101(9): 975–80.

[10] Haffner SM, Stern MP, Hazuda HP, et al. Cardiovascular risk factors in confirmed prediabetic individuals. Does the clock for coronary heart disease start ticking before the onset of clinical diabetes? JAMA 1990; 263:2893–8.

[11] Garvey WT, Kwon S, Zheng D, et al. Effects of insulin resistance and type 2 diabetes on lipoprotein subclass particle size and concentration determined by nuclear magnetic resonance. Diabetes 2003;52: 453–62.

[12] Austin MA, King MC, Vranizan KM, et al. Atherogenic lipoprotein phenotype. A proposed genetic marker for coronary heart disease risk. Circulation 1990;82:495–506.

[13] Austin MA, Breslow JL, Hennekens CH, et al. Low-density lipoprotein subclass patterns and risk of myocardial infarction. JAMA 1988;260:1917–21.

[14] Campos H, Genest Jr JJ, Blijlevens E, et al. Low density lipoprotein particle size and coronary artery disease. Arterioscler Thromb 1992;12:187–95.

[15] McNamara JR, Jenner JL, Li Z, et al. Change in LDL particle size is associated with change in plasma triglyceride concentration. Arteriosclerosis and Thrombosis 1992;12:1284–90.

[16] Berneis KK, Krauss RM. Metabolic origins and clinical significance of LDL heterogeneity. J Lipid Res 2002;43:1363–79.

[17] Hopkins GJ, Barter PJ. Role of triglyceride-rich lipoproteins and hepatic lipase in determining the particle size and composition of high density lipoproteins. J Lipid Res 1986;27:1265–77.

[18] Neel JV. Diabetes mellitus: a "thrifty" genotype rendered detrimental by "progress"? 1962. Bull World Health Organ 1999;77:694–703 [discussion: 692–3].

[19] Lee Y, Hirose H, Ohneda M, et al. Beta-cell lipotoxicity in the pathogenesis of non-insulin-dependent diabetes mellitus of obese rats: impairment in adipocyte-beta-cell relationships. Proc Natl Acad Sci U S A 1994;91:10878–82.

[20] Unger RH, Zhou YT. Lipotoxicity of beta-cells in obesity and in other causes of fatty acid spillover. Diabetes 2001;50(Suppl 1):S118–21.

[21] Listenberger LL, Ory DS, Schaffer JE. Palmitate-induced apoptosis can occur through a ceramide-independent pathway. J Biol Chem 2001;276: 14890–5.

[22] de Vries JE, Vork MM, Roemen TH, et al. Saturated but not mono-unsaturated fatty acids induce apoptotic cell death in neonatal rat ventricular myocytes. J Lipid Res 1997;38:1384–94.

[23] Cnop M, Hannaert JC, Hoorens A, et al. Inverse relationship between cytotoxicity of free fatty acids in pancreatic islet cells and cellular triglyceride accumulation. Diabetes 2001;50:1771–7.

[24] Shimabukuro M, Higa M, Zhou YT, et al. Lipoapoptosis in beta-cells of obese prediabetic fa/fa rats. Role of serine palmitoyltransferase over expression. J Biol Chem 1998;273:32487–90.

[25] Shimabukuro M, Ohneda M, Lee Y, et al. Role of nitric oxide in obesity-induced beta cell disease. J Clin Invest 1997;100:290–5.

[26] Hardy S, Langelier Y, Prentki M. Oleate activates phosphatidylinositol 3-kinase and promotes proliferation and reduces apoptosis of MDA-MB-231 breast cancer cells, whereas palmitate has opposite effects. Cancer Res 2000;60:6353–8.

[27] Ostrander DB, Sparagna GC, Amoscato AA, et al. Decreased cardiolipin synthesis corresponds with cytochrome c release in palmitate-induced cardiomyocyte apoptosis. J Biol Chem 2001;276:38061–7.

[28] Shimabukuro M, Wang MY, Zhou YT, et al.

Protection against lipoapoptosis of beta cells through leptin-dependent maintenance of Bcl- 2 expression. Proc Natl Acad Sci U S A 1998;95:9558–61.

[29] Maedler K, Spinas GA, Dyntar D, et al. Distinct effects of saturated and monounsaturated fatty acids on beta-cell turnover and function. Diabetes 2001;50: 69–76.

[30] Shimabukuro M, Zhou YT, Levi M, et al. Fatty acid-induced beta cell apoptosis: a link between obesity and diabetes. Proc Natl Acad Sci U S A 1998; 95:2498–502.

[31] Zhou YT, Grayburn P, Karim A, et al. Baetens lipo-toxic heart disease in obese rats: implications for human obesity. Proc Natl Acad Sci U S A 2000; 97:1784–9.

[32] Chu KC, Sohal RS, Sun SC, et al. Lipid cardiomy-opathy of the hypertrophied heart of gold thio-glucose obese mice. J Pathol 1969;97:99–103.

[33] Chien KR, Bellary A, Nicar M, et al. Induction of a reversible cardiac lipidosis by a dietary long-chain fatty acid (erucic acid). Relationship to lipid accumulation in border zones of myocardial infarcts. Am J Pathol 1983;112:68–77.

[34] Kelly DP, Hale DE, Rutledge SL, et al. Molecular basis of inherited medium-chain acyl-CoA dehydro-genase deficiency causing sudden child death. J Inherit Metab Dis 1992;15:171–80.

[35] Unger RH. The physiology of cellular liporegulation. Annu Rev Physiol 2003;65:333–47.

[36] Vincent HK, Powers SK, Dirks AJ, et al. Mechanism for obesity-induced increase in myocardial lipid peroxidation. Int J Obes Relat Metab Disord 2001; 25:378–88.

[37] Lin KT, Xue JY, Wong PY. Mechanisms of peroxy-nitrite-induced apoptosis in HL-60 cells. Adv Exp Med Biol 1999;469:569–75.

[38] Kim JB, Wright HM, Wright M, et al. ADD1/ SREBP1 activates PPAR gamma through the production of endogenous ligand. Proc Natl Acad Sci U S A 1998;95:4333–7.

[39] Kliewer SA, Forman BM, Blumberg B, et al. Differential expression and activation of a family of murine peroxisome proliferator-activated receptors. Proc Natl Acad Sci U S A 1994;91:7355–9.

[40] Schoonjans K, Staels B, Auwerx J. The peroxisome proliferator activated receptors (PPARS) and their effects on lipid metabolism and adipocyte differentiation. Biochim Biophys Acta 1996;1302(2): 10930–45.

[41] Zhou YT, Shimabukuro M, Wang MY, et al. Role of peroxisome proliferator –activated receptor alpha in disease of pancreatic beta cells. Proc Natl Acad Sci U S A 1998;95:8898–903.

[42] Bell DS. Heart failure: the frequent, forgotten, and often fatal complication of diabetes. Diabetes Care 2003;26(8):2433–41.

[43] Kawaguchi M, Asakura T, Saito F, et al. [Changes in diameter size and F-actin expression in the myocytes of patients with diabetes and streptozotocin-induced diabetes model rats]. J Cardiol 1999;34(6):333–9 [in Japanese].

[44] Schramm E, Wagner M, Nellessen U, et al. Ultra-structural changes of human cardiac atrial nerve endings in diabetes mellitus. Eur J Clin Invest 2000; 30(4):311–6.

[45] Anguera I, Magrina J, Setoain FJ, et al. [Anatomo-pathological bases of latent ventricular dysfunction in insulin-dependent diabetics]. Rev Esp Cardiol 1998;51:43–50 [in Spanish].

[46] Saito F, Kawaguchi M, Izumida J, et al. Alteration in haemodynamics and pathological changes in the cardiovascular system during the development of type 2 diabetes mellitus in OLETF rats. Diabetologia 2003;46:1161–9.

[47] Chen S, Evans T, Mukherjee K, et al. Diabetes-induced myocardial structural changes: role of endo-thelin-1 and its receptors. J Mol Cell Cardiol 2000; 32:1621–9.

[48] Hosking DJ, Bennett T, Hampton JR. Diabetic autonomic neuropathy. Diabetes 1978;27:1043–55.

[49] Gillon KR, King RH, Thomas PK. The pathology of diabetic neuropathy and the effects of aldose reductase inhibitors. Clin Endocrinol Metab 1986;15: 837–53.

[50] Adams Jr KF, Fonarow GC, Emerman CL, et al. Characteristics and outcomes of patients hospitalized for heart failure in the United States: rationale, design, and preliminary observations from the first 100,000 cases in the Acute Decompensated Heart Failure National Registry (ADHERE). Am Heart J 2005; 149:209–16.

[51] Stone PH, Muller JE, Hartwell T, et al. The effect of diabetes mellitus on prognosis and serial left ven-tricular function after acute myocardial infarction: contribution of both coronary disease and diastolic left ventricular dysfunction to the adverse prognosis. The MILIS Study Group. J Am Coll Cardiol 1989;14: 49–57.

[52] Ginsberg HN. Insulin resistance and cardiovascular disease. J Clin Invest 2000;106:453–8.

[53] Reaven GM, Lithell H, Landsberg L. Hypertension and associated metabolic abnormalities–the role of insulin resistance and the sympathoadrenal system. N Engl J Med 1996;334:374–81.

[54] Rubler S, Dlugash J, Yuceoglu YZ, et al. New type of cardiomyopathy associated with diabetic glomerulo-sclerosis. Am J Cardiol 1972;30:595–602.

[55] Giles TD, Sander GE. Myocardial disease in hyper-tensive-diabetic patients. Am J Med 1989;87(6A): 23S–8S.

[56] Iribarren C, Karter AJ, Go AS, et al. Glycemic control and heart failure among adult patients with diabetes. Circulation 2001;103:2668–73.

[57] Stratton IM, Adler AI, Neil HA, et al. Association of glycaemia with macrovascular and microvascular complications of type 2 diabetes (UKPDS 35): prospective observational study. BMJ 2000;321: 405–12.

[58] Nichols GA. Congestive heart failure in type 2 diabetes: prevalence, incidence, and risk factors. Diabetes Care 2001;24:1614–9.

[59] Collins R, Armitage J, Parish S, et al. Heart Protection Study Collaborative Group. MRC/BHF Heart Protection Study of cholesterol-lowering with simvastatin in 5963 people with diabetes: a randomised placebo-controlled trial. Lancet 2003;361: 2005–16.

[60] Colhoun HM, Betteridge DJ, Durrington PN, et al for CARDS investigators. Primary prevention of cardiovascular disease with atorvastatin in type 2 diabetes in the Collaborative Atorvastatin Diabetes Study (CARDS): multicentre randomised placebo-controlled trial. Lancet 2004;364:685–96.

[61] Cannon CP, Braunwald E, McCabe CH, et al for the Thrombolysis in Myocardial Infarction 22 Investigators. Intensive versus moderate lipid lowering with statins after acute coronary syndromes. N Engl J Med 2004;350:1495–504.

[62] LaRosa JC, Grundy SM, Waters DD, et al. Intensive lipid lowering with atorvastatin in patients with stable coronary disease. N Engl J Med 2005;352:1425–35.

[63] ALLHAT Officers and Coordinators for the ALLHAT Collaborative Research Group. The Antihypertensive and Lipid-Lowering Treatment to Prevent Heart Attack Trial. Major outcomes in moderately hypercholesterolemic, hypertensive patients randomized to pravastatin vs. usual care: The Antihypertensive and Lipid-Lowering Treatment to Prevent Heart Attack Trial (ALLHAT-LLT). JAMA 2002;288:2998–3007.

[64] Keech A, Simes RJ, Barter P, et al. Effects of long-term fenofibrate therapy on cardiovascular events in 9795 people with type 2 diabetes mellitus (the FIELD study): randomised controlled trial. Lancet 2003;366: 1846–61.

[65] Garg A, Grundy S. Nicotinic acid as therapy for dyslipidemia in non-insulin-dependent diabetes mellitus. JAMA 1990;264:723–6.

[66] Grundy SM, Vega GL, McGovern ME, et al. Efficacy, safety, and tolerability of once-daily niacin for the treatment of dyslipidemia associated with type 2 diabetes: results of the assessment of diabetes control and evaluation of the efficacy of Niaspan trial. Arch Intern Med 2002;162:1568–76.

[67] Tsalamandris C, Panagiotopoulos S, Sinha A, et al. Complementary effects of pravastatin and nicotinic acid in the treatment of combined hyperlipidaemia in diabetic and non-diabetic patients. J Cardiovasc Risk 1994;1:231–9.

[68] Elam MB, Hunninghake DB, Davis KB, et al. Effect of niacin on lipid and lipoprotein levels and glycemic control in patients with diabetes and peripheral arterial disease: the ADMIT study: A randomized trial. Arterial Disease Multiple Intervention Trial. JAMA 2000;284:1263–70.

[69] Haffner SM, for the American Diabetes Association. Dyslipidemia management in adults with diabetes. Diabetes Care 2004;(Suppl 1):S68–71.

[70] American Diabetes Association. Standards of medical care in diabetes. Diabetes Care 2005;28(Suppl 1): S4–36 [erratum: Diabetes Care 2005;28:990].

[71] Jiang R, Schulze MB, Li T, et al. Non-HDLcholesterol and apolipoprotein B predict cardiovascular disease events among men with type 2 diabetes. Diabetes Care 2004;27:1991–7.

[72] Lehto S, Ronnemaa T, Haffner SM, et al. Dyslipidemia and hyperglycemia predict coronary heart disease events in middle-aged patients with NIDDM. Diabetes 1997;46:1354–9.

[73] Lu W, Resnick HE, Jablonski KA, et al. Non-HDL cholesterol as a predictor of cardiovascular disease in type 2 diabetes: the Strong Heart Study. Diabetes Care 2003;26:16–23.

[74] Liu J, Sempos C, Donahue RP, et al. Joint distribution of non-HDL and LDL cholesterol and coronary heart disease risk prediction among individuals with and without diabetes. Diabetes Care 2005;28:1916–21.

[75] Jones PH, Davidson MH. Reporting rate of rhabdomyolysis with fenofibrate + statin versus gemfibrozil + any statin. Am J Cardiol 2005;95:120–2.

[76] DeFronzo RA, Goodman AM. Efficacy of metformin in patients with non-insulin-dependent diabetes mellitus. The Multicenter Metformin Study Group. N Engl J Med 1995;333:541–9.

[77] Fontbonne A, Charles MA, Juhan-Vague I, et al. The effect of metformin on the metabolic abnormalities associated with upper-body fat distribution. BIGPRO Study Group. Diabetes Care 1996;19:920–6.

[78] Aronoff S, Rosenblatt S, Braithwaite S, et al. Pioglitazone hydrochloride monotherapy improves glycemic control in the treatment of patients with type 2 diabetes: a 6-month randomized placebo-controlled dose-response study. The Pioglitazone 2001 Study Group. Diabetes Care 2000;23:1605–11.

[79] Horton ES, Whitehouse F, Ghazzi MN, et al. Troglitazone in combination with sulfonylurea restores glycemic control in patients with type 2 diabetes. The Troglitazone Study Group. Diabetes Care 1998;21: 1462–9.

[80] Fonseca V, Rosenstock J, Patwardhan R, et al. Effect of metformin and rosiglitazone combination therapy in patients with type 2 diabetes mellitus: a randomized controlled trial. JAMA 2000;283(13):1695–702 [erratum JAMA 2000;284:1384].

[81] Goldberg RB, Kendall DM, Deeg MA, et al. A comparison of lipid and glycemic effects of pioglitazone and rosiglitazone in patients with type 2 diabetes and dyslipidemia. Diabetes Care 2005;28: 1547–54.

[82] Dormandy JA, Charbonnel B, Eckland DJ, et al. Secondary prevention of macrovascular events in patients with type 2 diabetes in the PROactive Study (PROspective pioglitAzone Clinical Trial in macroVascular Events): a randomised controlled trial. Lancet 2005; 366:1279–89.

[83] Lewin AJ, Kipnes MS, Meneghini LF, et al. Simvastatin/Thiazolidinedione Study Group. Effects

of simvastatin on the lipid profile and attainment of low-density lipoprotein cholesterol goals when added to thiazolidinedione therapy in patients with type 2 diabetes mellitus: A multicenter, randomized, double-blind, placebo-controlled trial. Clin Ther 2004;26: 379–89.

[84] Ryan DH, Espeland MA, Foster GD, et al. (Action for Health in Diabetes): design and methods for a clinical trial of weight loss for the prevention of cardiovascular disease in type 2 diabetes. Control Clin Trials 2003;24:610–28.

[85] Fradkin J. Diabetes Clinical Trials: What Is New at NIDDK? Clinical Diabetes 2004;22:109–12.

[86] Downs JR, Clearfield M, Weiss S, et al. Primary prevention of acute coronary events with lovastatin in men and women with average cholesterol levels: results of AFCAPS/TexCAPS. Air Force/Texas Coronary Atherosclerosis Prevention Study. JAMA 1998; 279(20):1615–22.

[87] Sever PS, Dahlof B, Poulter NR, et al. Prevention of coronary and stroke events with atorvastatin in hypertensive patients who have average or lower-than-average cholesterol concentrations, in the Anglo-Scandinavian Cardiac Outcomes Trial–Lipid Lowering Arm (ASCOT-LLA): a multicentre randomized controlled trial. Lancet 2003;5(361):1149–58.

[88] Koskinen P, Manttari M, Manninen V, et al. Coronary heart disease incidence in NIDDM patients in the Helsinki Heart Study. Diabetes Care 1992;15:820–5.

[89] Shepherd J, Blauw GJ, Murphy MB, et al, Heart Protection Study Collaborative Group. MRC/BHF Heart Protection Study of cholesterol lowering with simvastatin in 20,536 high-risk individuals: a randomised placebo-controlled trial. Lancet 2002;360: 7–22.

[90] Pravastatin in elderly individuals at risk of vascular disease (PROSPER): a randomised controlled trial. Lancet 2002;360(9346):1623–30.

[91] Pyorala K, Pedersen TR, Kjekshus J, et al. Cholesterol lowering with simvastatin improves prognosis of diabetic patients with coronary heart disease. A subgroup analysis of the Scandinavian Simvastatin Survival Study (4S). Diabetes Care 1997; 20(4):614–20 [erratum: Diabetes Care 1997;20:1048].

[92] Sacks FM, Pfeffer MA, Moye LA, et al. The effect of pravastatin on coronary events after myocardial infarction in patients with average cholesterol levels. Cholesterol and Recurrent Events Trial investigators. N Engl J Med 1996;335:1001–9.

[93] The Long-Term Intervention with Pravastatin in Ischaemic Disease (LIPID) Study Group. Prevention of cardiovascular events and death with pravastatin in patients with coronary heart disease and a broad range of initial cholesterol levels. N Engl J Med 1998;339: 1349–57.

[94] Serruys PW, de Feyter P, Macaya C, et al. Fluvastatin for prevention of cardiac events following successful first percutaneous coronary intervention: a randomized controlled trial. JAMA 2002;287:3215–22.

[95] Hoogwerf BJ, Waness A, Cressman M, et al. Effects of aggressive cholesterol lowering and low-dose anticoagulation on clinical and angiographic outcomes in patients with diabetes: the Post Coronary Artery Bypass Graft Trial. Diabetes 1999;48: 1289–94.

[96] Rubins HB, Robins SJ, Collins D, et al. Gemfibrozil for the secondary prevention of coronary heart disease in men with low levels of high density lipoprotein cholesterol. Veterans Affairs High-Density Lipoprotein Cholesterol Intervention Trial Study Group. N Engl Med 1999;341:410–8.

[97] Rubins HB, Robins SJ, Collins D, et al. Diabetes, plasma insulin, and cardiovascular disease: subgroup analysis from the Department of Veterans Affairs high-density lipoprotein intervention trial (VA-HIT). Arch Intern Med 2002;162:2597–604.

ELSEVIER
SAUNDERS

Heart Failure Clin 2 (2006) 53 – 59

HEART
FAILURE
CLINICS

Albuminuria and Cardiovascular Risk

Zvezdana Bogojevic, MD, George L. Bakris, MD*

Rush University Medical Center, Chicago, IL, USA

Presence of chronic kidney disease (CKD) is a major public health concern around the world. It is an independent risk factor for cardiovascular (CV) morbidity and mortality [1,2]. In the United States, the incidence of end-stage renal disease (ESRD) has doubled since 1990 with an even larger population of individuals showing signs of kidney damage, particularly macroalbuminuria (proteinuria) [3]. Hypertension and macroalbuminuria are common diagnoses in patients who have ESRD and are starting maintenance dialysis. It is surmised that the majority of people who have CKD die from a CV event before reaching ESRD; heart failure and arrhythmia are the leading causes of death for patients within the first year of starting maintenance dialysis [3]. CKD is a cause and an effect of hypertension; it is present in 2% to 5% of patients who are hypertensive [4]. Treatment of hypertension with agents that achieve blood pressure (BP) goals and reduce proteinuria not only helps prevent or slow the progression of nephropathy but also reduce CV events [5,6]. The management of hypertension in CKD is challenging and generally requires a minimum of three different and complementary-acting antihypertensive medications to achieve the recommended BP goal of less than 130/80 mm Hg, as noted by national and international guidelines [2,7–9].

Epidemiology

The two most common causes of CKD are diabetes and hypertension [9]. CKD is divided into five stages based on glomerular filtration rate (GFR), beginning with GFR of less than 90 mL/min [4]. Macroalbuminuria (proteinuria) is indicative of kidney disease and is assessed with at least two different spot urine collections, taken within a few weeks of each other, that measure albumin and creatinine [10]. Persistent urinary albumin excretion between 30 and 299 mg of albumin per gram creatinine is defined as microalbuminuria, whereas macroalbuminuria is defined as greater than 300 mg of albumin per gram creatinine. Microalbuminuria may be transient and occurs in settings of any inflammatory process or infection that heralds fever, exercise, heart failure, and poor glycemic control [10]. Thus, any value obtained must be viewed in the context of a stable disease process and absence of the aforementioned factors; and testing should be repeated after a short time as per the new recommendations [10].

Microalbuminuria as a cardiovascular marker

Presence of microalbuminuria indicates generalized endothelial damage and increased vascular permeability secondary to inflammatory process or change in the vasculature, in general and specifically in the glomerular capillary wall [11,12]. Studies support the concept that microalbuminuria represents abnormal vascular responsiveness, as noted by a blunted vasodilator response and an increased risk for development of ischemic heart disease, an association that is independent of BP level [11,13]. Moreover,

* Corresponding author. Rush University Hypertension/ Clinical Research Center, Department of Preventive Medicine, Rush University Medical Center, 1700 West Van Buren Street, Suite 470, Chicago, IL 60612.

E-mail address: gbakris@earthlink.net (G.L. Bakris).

low serum albumin and the degree of albuminuria are important independent prognostic variables for CV events and can be used in addition to traditional coronary risk factors [14]. Macroalbuminuria correlates even more strongly with CV disease because of its association with other adverse risk factors, including hypertension, hypercholesterolemia, reduced high-density lipoproteins, increased intermediate density lipoproteins, and very low density lipoproteins [15,16]. Urinary protein excretion in postmenopausal women correlates with CV mortality independent of diabetes or hypertension [17]. In the Heart Outcomes Prevention Evaluation (HOPE) trial, the absolute degree of proteinuria was linked to a progressive increase in the relative risk for CV events and death [18]. A recent longitudinal cohort study in the Netherlands demonstrates a significant interaction among mean BP, risk for microalbuminuria, and levels of C-reactive protein [19].

Decreasing microalbuminuria during antihypertensive treatment decreases CV risk accordingly in an individual who is at the high range of microalbuminuria. The risk for developing serious CV events in hypertensive patients who have left ventricular hypertrophy increases significantly at a UACR level of ~1.2 mg/mmol [20]; and its reduction was associated with fewer CV events independent of BP [21]. Presence of microalbuminuria in apparently healthy individuals represents a systemic low-grade inflammation, may be used as a marker for CV risk, and could be combined with currently used highly sensitive C-reactive protein (CRP) [22]. Although isolated microalbuminuria represents a more benign condition and may have a better prognosis if present in patients who are hypertensive, treatment for CV prevention needs to be more aggressive. Microalbuminuria and high CRP levels are more frequent in metabolic syndrome, which could be complicated by BP elevation, as a complication of metabolic abnormalities. There is a greater than 100-fold higher risk of inflammatory microalbuminuria in obese patients who have concentric left ventricular hypertrophy than in lean patients who do not have left-ventricular hypertrophy. This finding may indicate that microalbuminuria combined with a low-grade inflammation might be used as a better prognostic factor than body size. This conclusion should have an evaluation in large-sample prospective studies [23].

Data from the Prevention of Renal and Vascular End-stage Disease (PREVEND) study demonstrated that atrial fibrillation is associated with microalbuminuria and an elevated CRP, independently of traditionally predisposed risk factors for atrial fibrillation.

This positive association was a fourfold higher when presence of microalbuminuria was accompanied by CRP, suggesting that influence of systemic inflammation and vascular dysfunction may play an important role in the etiology of atrial fibrillation [24]. The results from the European Diabetes Prospective Complications Study (EURODIAB PCS) also confirm that about 40% of patients who have type 1 diabetes with microalbuminuria progress to overt proteinuria [25]. The risk for development of clinical nephropathy may be especially high in those patients who have higher albumin excretion rate values, excess body fat, and inadequate metabolic control [25].

Monitoring of albuminuria should be an integrated part of hypertension management. If the level does not decline, the focus should be placed on altered treatment strategies to achieve the BP goal, as well as on adequate control of other risks factors [21]. Although prospective, controlled studies are necessary to assess the definitive role of microalbuminuria in CV outcome, the data thus far suggest that presence of microalbuminuria indicates an inflammatory process in the vasculature and serves as a marker similar to or in lieu of CRP to determine risk. Whereas to date only the Losartan Intervention For Endpoint Reduction (LIFE) trial has measured microalbuminuria prospectively and noted a better outcome with its reduction, meta-analyses of many trials dealing with CV events, all of which include heart failure, have shown a benefit of agents known to reduce microalbuminuria or macroalbuminuria and an increased incidence of kidney disease progression by those that lower pressure without affecting albuminuria [21,26–30]. Results of the definitive trial on the role of changes in albuminuria on CV risk will be in known in 2008 with the completion of the Avoiding Cardiovascular events through Combination therapy in Patients Living with Systolic Hypertension (ACCOMPLISH) trial [31].

Outcome trials and macroalbuminuria

According to the available study data, there is a significant correlation between the macroalbuminuria (proteinuria) level with kidney disease progression and CV mortality; reduction in the urinary protein excretion has been related to the delayed progression of renal dysfunction and a decline in CV events [29,32–34]. In the Reduction in Endpoints in Noninsulin dependent diabetes mellitus with the Angiotensin II Antagonist Losartan (RENAAL) study, patients who had a high baseline albuminuria (>3 g/g creatinine) had a 1.92-fold higher risk for developing the CV endpoint and a 2.70-fold higher risk for heart failure when compared with those who had low albuminuria at the baseline (<1.5 g/g creatinine). Reduction in albuminuria during a 6-month period was correlated with CV risk reduction: For every 50% reduction in albuminuria there was an 18% reduction in CV risk and a 27% reduction in heart failure risk [29]. Worsening of albuminuria paralleled an increase in CV complications, as demonstrated in a several retrospective and prospective trials.

For determination of renal function deterioration, level of proteinuria was more relevant than baseline level of GFR in the African-American Study of Kidney Disease (AASK) [32]. In a separate trial of nondiabetic kidney disease progression, this observation was confirmed. In the COOPERATE (combination treatment of antiotensin II receptor blocker [ARB] and angiotensin converting enzyme [ACE] inhibitor in nondiabetic renal disease) study, there was a significant delay to ESRD in the group that received a combination of an ARB and ACE inhibitor compared with either monotherapy. The improved outcomes of the combination have little to do with BP differences and everything to do with differences in proteinuria (Fig. 1) [35]. Thus, the additive

antiproteinuric effects of this antiproteinuric combination, attributed to the renin-angiotensin-aldosterone system blockade, could increase renal survival [36].

Interventions of the earlier stages of CKD and of related CV risk factors (anemia, hypertension, dyslipidemia) can be effective in reducing the progression to kidney failure as well as in preventing the consequent systemic CV complications [37–39]. Thus, based on current recommendations and results of trials, to delay deterioration of the kidney function as well as CKD progression, antihypertensive treatment should be aimed at not only reducing BP but also at preventing increases in microalbuminuria and reducing pre-existing levels of proteinuria. Not all agents are equal in their effects, however. Moreover, even antihypertensive agents that blunt the renin-angiotensin-aldosterone system can be limited by patients' ingesting of a high sodium diet [40].

Antihypertensive agents and albuminuria reduction

ACE inhibitors and ARBs attenuate increases in albuminuria by their effects in the glomerulus on angiotensin II and the autoregulation of the GFR [6,41]. In the Angiotensin-converting-enzyme Inhibition in Progressive Renal Insufficiency (AIPRI) trial,

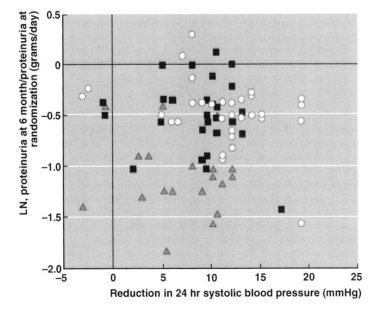

Fig. 1. Change in 24-hour ambulatory blood pressure measurement and proteinuria at 6 months in the COOPERATE Trial. (*Adapted from* Nakao N, Seno H, Kasuga H, et al. Effects of combination treatment with losartan and trandolapril on office and ambulatory blood pressures in non-diabetic renal disease: A COOPERATE-ABP substudy. Am J Nephrol 2004;24(5): 543–8; with permission.)

patients randomized to the ACE inhibitor benazepril achieved a greater improvement in renal function compared with placebo, with a 66% risk reduction in the disease progression [42]. In the Ramipril Efficacy in Nephropathy (REIN) trial of nondiabetic renal disease patients who had serum creatinine values of greater than 177 μmol/L (2.0 mg/dL) and greater than 3.0 g/d of proteinuria had a 62% reduction in renal disease progression, whereas those with microalbuminuria had only a 22% reduction in renal disease progression over the same 42-month follow-up [43]. Similarly, African Americans [26] have a higher likelihood of developing progressive renal disease and derive additional renoprotection from blockade of the renin-angiotensin-aldosterone system. In the AASK trial, the primary endpoint was the rate of change in GFR (GFR slope), clinical composite outcome of reduction in GFR by 50% or more (or ≥25 mL/min per 1.73 m^2) from baseline, ESRD, or death. The ramipril group manifested risk reductions in the clinical composite outcome of 22% (95% CI, 1%–38%; $P = .04$) and 38% (95% CI, 14%–56%; $P = .004$) when compared with the metoprolol and amlodipine groups, respectively [44]. Prognostic signs that correlate with a delay in CKD progression include goal BP less than 130/80 mm Hg or a 30% increase in serum creatinine (baseline <3 mg/dL) within the first 4 months of therapy and a reduction of greater than 30% from baseline levels of proteinuria [8].

Because of their excellent tolerability and proven efficacy, these agents should be up-titrated unless contraindicated by hyperkalemia (serum [K+] >5.5 mEq/L). Maximal approved BP lowering doses are preferred because of their benefit at these dosages in clinical trials. Dose-titration beyond BP control for maximal proteinuria reduction has been advocated as a strategy to optimize CV risk, especially in patients who have diabetes [45–47].

Salt restriction and pretreatment with a diuretic can increase the response of renin-angiotensin-aldosterone system blockers [48], especially in African Americans [49], and thus improve the BP and optimally reduce proteinuria. In fact, increased salt intake significantly blunts the antihypertensive effect of all agents except for calcium antagonists.

Calcium antagonists (CAs) have not been studied extensively in nephropathy, although two prospective randomized trials clearly demonstrate that dihydropyridine CAs have much less effect on slowing kidney disease progression in those who have proteinuria and advanced disease than blockers of the renin-angiotensin-aldosterone system. This outcome is well illustrated by a recent systematic review of the data and perspective on CA use in people who have proteinuria [27,50]. Moreover, the National Kidney Foundation guidelines state that their use is relatively contraindicated unless coincident with a blocker of the renin-angiotensin-aldosterone system [8]. Nondihydropyridine agents, such as verapamil and diltiazem, are much more efficacious in lowering proteinuria in advanced disease; but all agents are similar in patients who have microalbuminuria, if BP is reduced [27,51].

Beta blockers are recognized as useful adjunctive therapy for patients who have CKD, and they have been shown in some trials to lower proteinuria by a similar magnitude to ACE inhibitors in patients who are not diabetic [52]. Newer agents like carvedilol, however, reduce CV mortality and microalbuminuria development without adversely affecting glucose tolerance or lipid profiles [53].

Recommendations

Evidence indicates that patients who have microalbuminuria are just as likely to die from CV disease as they are to progress to ESRD. Populations at risk for CKD (diabetes, hypertension, or family history) should be screened annually for microalbuminuria. Documented persistent elevations (two out of three measurements above reference range) in individuals undergoing treatment for elevated BP, lipid disorders, or both, should be retested within 6 months (Fig. 2). After diagnosis and evaluation, continued surveillance is recommended to assess progression of renal disease and response to therapy. Agents that block the renin-angiotensin-aldosterone system (ACE inhibitors and ARBs) are preferred initial therapy because of their favorable effects on BP and albuminuria. Because of their widespread tolerability, they can be dose-titrated for maximal proteinuria reduction (Fig. 3). Diuretics can potentiate the effects of ACE inhibitors and ARBs. Nondihydropyridine CAs are superior to dihydropyridine CAs in proteinuria reduction despite the similar BP–lowering effects.

Macroalbuminuria (proteinuria) as well as microalbuminuria are plausible targets to watch as BP is being lowered toward the goal. It is clear that lowering of BP alone without lowering urine protein does not result in optimal kidney outcomes, but the CV outcomes in this context have never been evaluated. Evaluation of albuminuria changes in the context of CV outcomes is the focus of ongoing clinical trials to be completed within the next four years.

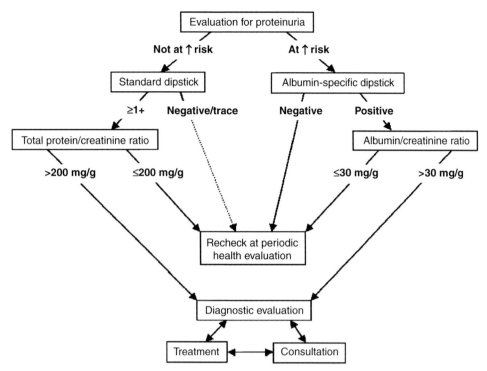

Fig. 2. Evaluation and work-up of microalbuminuria. (*Adapted from* the National Kidney Foundation Guidelines.) (*From* Clinical practice recommendations 2005. Diabetes Care 2005;28(Suppl 1):S1–79; with permission.)

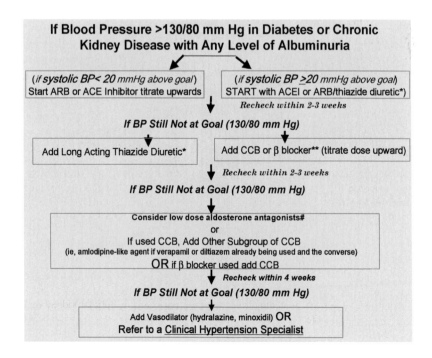

Fig. 3. An approach to achieving blood pressure goals in the patient who has albuminuria with or without kidney disease or diabetes. ACEI, angiotensin-converting enzyme inhibitor; CCB, calcium channel blocker.

References

[1] Manjunath G, Tighiouart H, Ibrahim H, et al. Level of kidney function as a risk factor for atherosclerotic cardiovascular outcomes in the community. J Am Coll Cardiol 2003;41(1):47–55.

[2] Chobanian AV, Bakris GL, Black HR, et al. Seventh report of the Joint National Committee on Prevention, Detection, Evaluation, and Treatment of High Blood Pressure. Hypertension 2003;42(6):1206–52.

[3] United States Renal Data System. Available at: http://www.USRDS.org. Accessed September 15, 2005.

[4] K/DOQI clinical practice guidelines for chronic kidney disease: evaluation, classification, and stratification. Kidney Disease Outcome Quality Initiative. Am J Kidney Dis 2002;39(2, Suppl 2):S1–246.

[5] Chua DC, Bakris GL. Is proteinuria a plausible target of therapy? Curr Hypertens Rep 2004;6(3):177–81.

[6] Bakris G. Proteinuria and blood pressure reduction: are they of equal importance to preserve kidney function? Curr Hypertens Rep 2005;7(5):357–8.

[7] 2003 European Society of Hypertension-European Society of Cardiology guidelines for the management of arterial hypertension. J Hypertens 2003;21(6):1011–53.

[8] K/DOQI clinical practice guidelines on hypertension and antihypertensive agents in chronic kidney disease. Am J Kidney Dis 2004;43(5, Suppl 2):1–290.

[9] Clinical practice recommendations 2005. Diabetes Care 2005;28(Suppl 1):S1–79.

[10] Eknoyan G, Hostetter T, Bakris GL, et al. Proteinuria and other markers of chronic kidney disease: a position statement of the National Kidney Foundation (NKF) and the National Institute of Diabetes and Digestive and Kidney Diseases (NIDDK). Am J Kidney Dis 2003;42(4):617–22.

[11] Garg JP, Bakris GL. Microalbuminuria: marker of vascular dysfunction, risk factor for cardiovascular disease. Vasc Med 2002;7(1):35–43.

[12] Russo LM, Bakris GL, Comper WD. Renal handling of albumin: a critical review of basic concepts and perspective. Am J Kidney Dis 2002;39(5):899–919.

[13] Clausen P, Jensen JS, Jensen G, et al. Elevated urinary albumin excretion is associated with impaired arterial dilatory capacity in clinically healthy subjects. Circulation 2001;103(14):1869–74.

[14] Anavekar NS, Gans DJ, Berl T, et al. Predictors of cardiovascular events in patients with type 2 diabetic nephropathy and hypertension: a case for albuminuria. Kidney Int Suppl 2004;(92):S50–5.

[15] Sibley SD, Hokanson JE, Steffes MW, et al. Increased small dense LDL and intermediate-density lipoprotein with albuminuria in type 1 diabetes. Diabetes Care 1999;22(7):1165–70.

[16] Bianchi S, Bigazzi R, Campese VM. Microalbuminuria in essential hypertension: significance, pathophysiology, and therapeutic implications. Am J Kidney Dis 1999;34(6):973–95.

[17] Roest M, Banga JD, Janssen WM, et al. Excessive urinary albumin levels are associated with future cardiovascular mortality in postmenopausal women. Circulation 2001;103(25):3057–61.

[18] Gerstein HC, Mann JF, Yi Q, et al. Albuminuria and risk of cardiovascular events, death, and heart failure in diabetic and nondiabetic individuals. JAMA 2001;286(4):421–6.

[19] Stuveling EM, Bakker SJ, Hillege HL, et al. C-reactive protein modifies the relationship between blood pressure and microalbuminuria. Hypertension 2004;43(4):791–6.

[20] Ibsen H, Wachtell K, Olsen MH, et al. Albuminuria and cardiovascular risk in hypertensive patients with left ventricular hypertrophy: the LIFE Study. Kidney Int 2004;65(92 Suppl):S56–8.

[21] Ibsen H, Olsen MH, Wachtell K, et al. Reduction in albuminuria translates to reduction in cardiovascular events in hypertensive patients: losartan intervention for endpoint reduction in hypertension study. Hypertension 2005;45(2):198–202.

[22] Nakamura M, Onoda T, Itai K, et al. Association between serum C-reactive protein levels and microalbuminuria: a population-based cross-sectional study in northern Iwate, Japan. Intern Med 2004;43(10):919–25.

[23] Pedrinelli R, Dell'Omo G, Di B, et al. Low-grade inflammation and microalbuminuria in hypertension. Arterioscler Thromb Vasc Biol 2004;24(12):2414–9.

[24] Asselbergs FW, van den Berg MP, Diercks GF, et al. C-reactive protein and microalbuminuria are associated with atrial fibrillation. Int J Cardiol 2005;98(1):73–7.

[25] Giorgino F, Laviola L, Cavallo PP, et al. Factors associated with progression to macroalbuminuria in microalbuminuric type 1 diabetic patients: the EURODIAB Prospective Complications Study. Diabetologia 2004;47(6):1020–8.

[26] Vaur L, Gueret P, Lievre M, et al. Development of congestive heart failure in type 2 diabetic patients with microalbuminuria or proteinuria: observations from the DIABHYCAR (type 2 DIABetes, Hypertension, CArdiovascular Events and Ramipril) study. Diabetes Care 2003;26(3):855–60.

[27] Nathan S, Pepine CJ, Bakris GL. Calcium antagonists. effects on cardio-renal risk in hypertensive patients. Hypertension 2005;46:637–42.

[28] Mann JF, Gerstein HC, Pogue J, et al. Renal insufficiency as a predictor of cardiovascular outcomes and the impact of ramipril: the HOPE randomized trial. Ann Intern Med 2001;134(8):629–36.

[29] De Zeeuw D, Remuzzi G, Parving HH, et al. Albuminuria, a therapeutic target for cardiovascular protection in type 2 diabetic patients with nephropathy. Circulation 2004;110:921–7.

[30] Berl T, Hunsicker LG, Lewis JB, et al. Impact of achieved blood pressure on cardiovascular outcomes in the Irbesartan Diabetic Nephropathy Trial. J Am Soc Nephrol 2005;16(7):2170–9.

[31] Jamerson KA, Bakris GL, Wun CC, et al. Rationale and design of the avoiding cardiovascular events

through combination therapy in patients living with systolic hypertension (ACCOMPLISH) trial: the first randomized controlled trial to compare the clinical outcome effects of first-line combination therapies in hypertension. Am J Hypertens 2004;17(9):793–801.

[32] Lea J, Greene T, Hebert L, et al. The relationship between magnitude of proteinuria reduction and risk of end-stage renal disease: results of the African American study of kidney disease and hypertension. Arch Intern Med 2005;165(8):947–53.

[33] De Zeeuw D, Remuzzi G, Parving HH, et al. Proteinuria, a target for renoprotection in patients with type 2 diabetic nephropathy: lessons from RENAAL. Kidney Int 2004;65(6):2309–20.

[34] Pohl MA, Blumenthal S, Cordonnier DJ, et al. Independent and additive impact of blood pressure control and angiotensin II receptor blockade on renal outcomes in the Irbesartan Diabetic Nephropathy Trial: clinical implications and limitations. J Am Soc Nephrol 2005; 16(10):3027–37.

[35] Nakao N, Seno H, Kasuga H, et al. Effects of combination treatment with losartan and trandolapril on office and ambulatory blood pressures in non-diabetic renal disease: A COOPERATE-ABP substudy. Am J Nephrol 2004;24(5):543–8.

[36] Nakao N, Yoshimura A, Morita H, et al. Combination treatment of angiotensin-II receptor blocker and angiotensin-converting-enzyme inhibitor in non-diabetic renal disease (COOPERATE): a randomised controlled trial. Lancet 2003;361(9352):117–24.

[37] Estacio RO, Jeffers BW, Gifford N, et al. Effect of blood pressure control on diabetic microvascular complications in patients with hypertension and type 2 diabetes. Diabetes Care 2000;23(Suppl 2):B54–64.

[38] Schrier RW, Estacio RO, Esler A, et al. Effects of aggressive blood pressure control in normotensive type 2 diabetic patients on albuminuria, retinopathy and strokes. Kidney Int 2002;61(3):1086–97.

[39] Gaede P, Vedel P, Larsen N, et al. Multifactorial intervention and cardiovascular disease in patients with type 2 diabetes. N Engl J Med 2003;348(5):383–93.

[40] Bakris GL, Weir MR. Salt intake and reductions in arterial pressure and proteinuria. Is there a direct link? Am J Hypertens 1996;9(12 Pt 2):200S–6S.

[41] Bakris GL, Stein JH. Diabetic nephropathy. Dis Mon 1993;39(8):573–611.

[42] Maschio G, Alberti D, Janin G, et al. Effect of the angiotensin-converting-enzyme inhibitor benazepril on the progression of chronic renal insufficiency. The Angiotensin-Converting-Enzyme Inhibition in Progressive Renal Insufficiency Study Group. N Engl J Med 1996;334(15):939–45.

[43] The GISEN Group (Gruppo Italiano di Studi Epidemiologici in Nefrologia). Randomised placebo-controlled trial of effect of ramipril on decline in glomerular filtration rate and risk of terminal renal failure in proteinuric, non-diabetic nephropathy. Lancet 1997;349(9069):1857–63.

[44] Wright Jr JT, Bakris G, Greene T, et al. Effect of blood pressure lowering and antihypertensive drug class on progression of hypertensive kidney disease: results from the AASK trial. JAMA 2002;288(19):2421–31.

[45] Weinberg MS, Kaperonis N, Bakris GL. How high should an ACE inhibitor or angiotensin receptor blocker be dosed in patients with diabetic nephropathy? Curr Hypertens Rep 2003;5(5):418–25.

[46] Peters H, Ritz E. Dosing angiotensin II blockers– beyond blood pressure. Nephrol Dial Transplant 1999; 14(11):2568–70.

[47] Bakris GL, Slataper R, Vicknair N, et al. ACE inhibitor mediated reductions in renal size and microalbuminuria in normotensive, diabetic subjects. J Diabetes Complications 1994;8(1):2–6.

[48] Buter H, Hemmelder MH, Navis G, et al. The blunting of the antiproteinuric efficacy of ACE inhibition by high sodium intake can be restored by hydrochlorothiazide. Nephrol Dial Transplant 1998;13(7):1682–5.

[49] Douglas JG, Bakris GL, Epstein M, et al. Management of high blood pressure in African Americans: consensus statement of the Hypertension in African Americans Working Group of the International Society on Hypertension in Blacks. Arch Intern Med 2003; 163(5):525–41.

[50] Bakris GL, Weir MR, Secic M, et al. Differential effects of calcium antagonist subclasses on markers of nephropathy progression. Kidney Int 2004;65(6): 1991–2002.

[51] Ruggenenti P, Fassi A, Ilieva AP, et al. Preventing microalbuminuria in type 2 diabetes. N Engl J Med 2004;351(19):1941–51.

[52] Agodoa LY, Appel L, Bakris GL, et al. Effect of ramipril vs. amlodipine on renal outcomes in hypertensive nephrosclerosis: a randomized controlled trial. JAMA 2001;285(21):2719–28.

[53] Bakris GL, Fonseca V, Katholi RE, et al. Metabolic effects of carvedilol vs. metoprolol in patients with type 2 diabetes mellitus and hypertension: a randomized controlled trial. JAMA 2004;292(18):2227–36.

ELSEVIER
SAUNDERS

Heart Failure Clin 2 (2006) 61 – 70

HEART
FAILURE
CLINICS

The Effect of Hyperglycemia and Its Therapies on the Heart

Kathleen L. Wyne, MD, PhD, FACE*

University of Texas Southwestern Medical Center at Dallas, Dallas, TX, USA

Diabetes mellitus (DM) has been identified as a risk factor for morbidity and mortality in heart failure. Although DM is a clear risk factor for the development of heart failure, the incidence of DM in patients who have heart failure is increased markedly above that of the general population. These observations lead to questions regarding the role of diabetes in the cause of heart failure. Epidemiologic studies have shown that persons with type 1 or type 2 DM are at increased risk of all forms of cardiovascular disease (CVD) affecting the heart, brain, and peripheral blood vessels [1–4]. The excess risk of both subclinical atherosclerosis and CVD actually begins in states of abnormal glucose regulation, including impaired fasting glucose (IFG), impaired glucose tolerance (IGT), and insulin resistance [5–8]. The slow, insidious development of the macrovascular and microvascular complications related to diabetes contribute to the fact that people with diabetes usually are not diagnosed with CVD until they have very extensive disease, and often their symptoms, which may be vague and nonspecific, are not recognized as manifestations of CVD [8–12].

Clinical studies designed to prevent the complications of diabetes have shown that improving the hyperglycemia prevents microvascular events but not macrovascular events [13,14]. One exception has been the overweight subgroup in the UKPDS study [15], in which treatment with metformin was associated with a statistically significant decrease in myo-

cardial infarctions, but the significance of this observation is unknown. Treatment of insulin resistance in patients who have established diabetes and vascular disease was found recently not to have a statistically significant decrease in the composite vascular endpoint [16]. The long-term observation, over a mean of 17 years, of the Diabetes Control and Complications Trial [17] cohort has shown that 6.5 years of intensive glucose control has delayed benefits in preventing macrovascular disease in patients who have type 1 diabetes. Given the long duration of time required to see this benefit in people with type 1 diabetes, it is possible that the window of opportunity has already been lost when type 2 diabetes is diagnosed because most of these people have had a prolonged period of hyperglycemia before they were diagnosed. Studies are now ongoing toward understanding the vasculature changes and developing therapies that will be effective once the hyperglycemia is diagnosed. Simultaneously, strategies are being developed to diagnose type 2 diabetes earlier in the disease process to prevent the morbidity and mortality associated with the disease.

The metabolic changes associated with insulin resistance, abnormal glucose regulation, and ultimately hyperglycemia, that are used to identify type 2 diabetes begin long before the serum glucose level is elevated. This is likely why the studies designed to prevent complications associated with diabetes have not been very successful [13–15,18]. Animal studies have shown that there are abnormalities in fat metabolism that begin long before the serum glucose level rises, which lead to an elevation of circulating free fatty acids (FFAs) [19], leading to the production of inflammatory cytokines, which are initially involved in local changes in the vasculature in the adipose tissue. Over time, the excess free fatty acids are de-

---

* Division of Endocrinology and Metabolism, Department of Internal Medicine, University of Texas Southwestern Medical Center at Dallas, 5323 Harry Hines Boulevard, Dallas, TX 75390-8857.

E-mail address: Kathleen.Wyne@UTSouthwestern.edu

posited in nonadipose tissues, a process that has been termed ectopic fat deposition, which leads to lipotoxicity [20,21]. This ectopic fat deposition can lead to abnormal cell function and, potentially, to cell death but also can result in further inappropriate production of inflammatory cytokines, thus exacerbating the miscommunication between the vasculature and the adipose tissue. At the same time, hyperglycemia leads to the glycation of cell proteins, thereby altering the function of vascular endothelial cells, vascular smooth muscle cells, and cardiomyocytes, which leads to a decrease in contractility and an increase in inflammatory cytokines. The hyperlipidemia that is typically present in the presence of insulin resistance or uncontrolled hyperglycemia provides another mechanism for increasing inflammation and altering vascular function. The elevations in glucose, free fatty acids, lipids, and cytokines together lead to abnormal vascular function and, ultimately, heart failure. As the age at which diabetes has been found has decreased, the age at which heart failure occurs is also decreasing.

Lipotoxicity

Free fatty acids

The metabolic abnormalities that occur in the adipose tissue are a combination of environmental (ie, excess delivery of nutrients for storage) and genetic factors (ie, an inability to store or metabolize the excess of nutrients). Although a healthy lifestyle is one proven method for preventing this process, people appear to have different levels of sensitivity for developing the early stages of lipotoxicity. As the adipocyte enlarges while trying to store the excess nutrients, it also tries to metabolize excess nutrients to minimize the mechanical stress on the cell. These changes, in addition to the intracellular energy fluxes, disrupt cellular homeostasis and lead to intracellular stress responses. One of these responses, the endoplasmic reticulum (ER) stress response, occurs when the intracellular stress alters the homeostasis in the endoplasmic reticulum, leading to the activation of a signal transduction system linking the ER lumen with the cytoplasm and nucleus. Intracellular signaling pathways are then activated or deactivated, leading to alterations in the activity of enzymes such as AMP-kinase and the c-Jun N-terminal kinase, which then affects the phosphorylation status of the insulin receptor and IRS-1, thus facilitating insulin resistance in the cell [22]. Insulin is then not able to activate its receptor to prevent lipolysis, and the unregulated release of FFAs

results in an alteration of the circulating levels of the adipose-derived cytokines (also called adipocytokines). These cytokines include adiponectin, leptin, tumor necrosis factor (TNF)-α, interleukin (IL)-6, and resistin. The enlarged adipocytes then secrete less adiponectin and more leptin and TNF-α as a form of communication to the nonadipose tissues to stimulate fatty acid oxidation, thus depleting the whole body load of fatty acids. TNF-α also stimulates preadipocytes to produce monocyte chemoattractant protein (MCP)-1. The local endothelial cells respond by also secreting MCP-1. The increased secretion of leptin by the adipocytes also stimulates the transport of macrophages to adipose tissue. The decreased production of adiponectin by adipocytes may also contribute to the adhesion of macrophages to endothelial cells. Once these cells are activated, they contribute to perpetuating a vicious cycle of macrophage recruitment, production of inflammatory cytokines, and impairment of adipocyte function, which results in alterations in insulin action [23]. Consequently, the altered pattern of adipocytokines, which were probably generated originally as a protective mechanism, initiate an inflammatory process that affects the endothelium throughout the body and the nonadipose tissues.

Inflammation

Epidemiologic studies have shown that markers of inflammation predict a risk for vascular disease, hypertension, and type 2 diabetes. The processes by which inflammation affects the pathogenesis of vascular disease are under intense study. The insulin resistance that is present in type 2 diabetes contributes to the inflammation and may actually be a causal factor. The mechanisms that initiate inflammation in type 1 diabetes are not yet clear. Hyperglycemia alone does not appear to be sufficient because not all patients who have uncontrolled type 1 diabetes have elevated markers of inflammation. Data from the Pittsburgh Epidemiology of Diabetes Complications (EDC) Study [24] have shown that higher adiponectin levels are associated prospectively with a lower risk of coronary artery disease (CAD) in people who have type 1 diabetes, suggesting that the underlying mechanisms may be the same and could be unrelated to the glucose. Recent prospective data from this study have shown that blood pressure, lipid levels, inflammatory markers, renal disease, and peripheral vascular disease showed a positive gradient across the groups consisting of no CAD, angina, and hard CAD, whereas glycosylated hemoglobin (HbA$_{1c}$) showed no association with subsequent CAD

[10,25]. In addition to lipotoxicity, it is possible that the vascular damage found in type 1 diabetes is the result of the direct effects of glucose and lipids through oxidative stress. Further studies are needed to evaluate the vascular disease in people with type 1 diabetes, especially those who have elevated markers of inflammation. Additionally, studies are needed to ascertain whether there are plaque differences in patients who have type 1 and type 2 diabetes. The relationship among risk factors, plaque characteristics, and the natural history of the atherosclerosis between the two types of diabetes will help to determine whether glucose plays a role in the inflammation and, if it does, whether it is primary or secondary in the cause of the vascular disease.

Glucose toxicity

Advanced glycation end products and receptors for advanced glycation end products

In the presence of any amount of hyperglycemia, nonenzymatic glycoxidation of proteins and lipids leads to the formation of a series of products that are referred to collectively as advanced glycation end products (AGEs) [26,27]. The advanced glycation end products are the result of a nonenzymatic reaction of reducing glucose with primary amino groups of proteins called the Maillard reaction. AGEs have been shown to act directly to induce protein cross-links, which are protease resistant and cause irreversible damage to cells and tissues. Through cell surface receptors, such as the receptors for AGEs (RAGE), AGEs also induce the release of cytokines, which leads to the activation of cells such as monocytes and macrophages, vascular smooth muscles cells, and endothelial cells, resulting in the production of reactive oxygen species (ROS) that induce the oxidation of DNA and peroxidation of membrane lipids [28]. The inhibition of RAGE is associated with an attenuation of diabetes-associated atherosclerosis in animal models [29]. An endogenous, soluble truncated form of RAGE (esRAGE) has been found that apparently functions to bind circulating AGEs and neutralize them [30].

The inability of the body to clear the AGEs contributes both direct toxicity to the vessel walls and indirect toxicity through the ability of AGEs to increase inflammatory cytokines. The direct effect is one of pure mechanical dysfunction caused by AGE cross-bridges established between macromolecules. This prevents the structural proteins from moving properly during vascular contraction and dilation, thus

transforming vessel walls into stiff, inelastic tubes and disturbing basement membrane adhesion properties. In the case of cardiomyocytes, the effect of the AGEs is to decrease contractility. This condition will result in high blood pressure, leaky vessels, and in the case of the heart, stiffness in the form of diastolic dysfunction. AGE accumulation will also damage the blood vessels by trapping proteins (eg, immunoglobulins and lipoproteins) and cells in the vessel walls, thus stimulating the immune and inflammatory response that has been described in atherosclerosis.

The pathways that may be affected by the binding of AGEs to the cell surface RAGEs include the generation of inflammatory cytokines and growth factors, thus leading to intimal proliferation and an overproduction of extracellular matrix, which may also contribute to the stiffness of the vessel. This process could possibly then be exacerbated by the events occurring in the adipose tissue, the presence of oxidized lipoproteins, and perhaps, either viral or bacterial infectious events. The constitutive presence of AGE receptors on resting T lymphocytes (CD4 and CD8) has led to the hypothesis that their activation in the vessel wall may trigger a low-grade, sustained inflammatory state, which could be accelerated by any elevation in glucose above the normal range. Consequently, the changes in the vasculature begin in all states of abnormal glucose regulation, including impaired fasting glucose (IFG), impaired glucose tolerance (IGT), and insulin resistance. Thus, it is not surprising that epidemiologic studies have shown that the excess risk of both subclinical atherosclerosis and CVD actually begins before the diagnosis of diabetes and before the diagnosis of "prediabetes."

Oxidative stress

The observation that a long duration of elevated glucose is required for the development in some but not all people who have type 1 DM raises the question of what, other than glucose, contributes to the excess vascular disease. Certainly, the glycation of proteins in the vascular wall can alter vascular function, but hyperglycemia alone does not account for all of the clinically relevant vascular disease. Some but not all studies have shown that lipid abnormalities account for some of the cardiovascular risk in type 1 diabetes. Recent data from three studies of people who have type 1 diabetes have shown that lipid parameters do predict cardiovascular risk; however, the studies have conflicting data as to which parameters [10,31,32]. Nonetheless, lipid parameters remain stronger predictors of risk than chronic hyperglycemia. Studies of lipid metabolism have shown that hyperlipidemia is associated with increased lipid oxidation and oxidative stress.

Oxidative stress refers to an imbalance in the ability of a tissue to generate ROS (ie, superoxide anions $[O_2^-]$, hydrogen peroxide $[H_2O_2]$, peroxynitrite $[ONOO^-]$, and hydroxyl radicals $[OH^-]$) and to eliminate them through enzymatic (ie, through superoxide dismutase, catalase, and glutathione peroxidase) or nonenzymatic (ie, glutathione and vitamins C and E) systems. Oxidative stress occurs when ROS production overrides the metabolic capacity of the antioxidant defense system. This excess of ROS results typically in tissue damage. The excess production of ROS can cause further damage through the use of nitric oxide (NO). Nitric oxide plays a role in maintaining the health of many cellular functions through its ability to donate electrons to transition metals, especially the iron moiety of soluble guanylyl cyclase. Endogenous inhibitors of nitric oxide, such as asymmetric dimethylarginine (ADMA) may also contribute to the generation of oxidative stress. Consequently, any disease state that leads to a reduced antioxidant defense system can have tissue damage caused by excess ROS or oxidative stress. Hyperlipidemia and hyperglycemia have both been shown to increase ROS generation. Additionally, decreased levels of antioxidants and of ADMA have been described in diabetes. The increase in oxidative stress (ie, excess production of ROS) activates macrophages and endothelial cells, thus leading to inflammation and abnormal endothelial function. The oxidative stress will also facilitate damage to the cardiomyocyte, leading to decreased contractility, fibrosis, and ultimately to heart failure.

Most, if not all, risk factors related to atherosclerosis and CV morbidity and mortality, including traditional and nontraditional risk factors, are also found to be associated with endothelial dysfunction [33]. Endothelial dysfunction is characterized by impaired endothelium-dependent vasodilation, which is caused by a reduction of the bioavailability of vasodilators, NO in particular, and endothelial activation, which is characterized by a proinflammatory, proliferative, and procoagulatory milieu that favors all stages of atherogenesis [34]. In addition to the increased oxidative stress, hyperinsulinemia, similar to that observed in insulin-resistant individuals after an overnight fast, causes severe endothelial dysfunction, which has been proposed to be a result of increased oxidant stress. The inappropriate elevation of plasma FFA as seen in insulin resistance is associated with endothelial dysfunction [35–37]. Several mechanisms have been proposed by which FFA could influence endothelium-dependent vasodilation. Plasma FFA

elevation lowers circulating levels of most amino acids, including L-arginine, which may reduce the substrate for NO formation [38]. The direct inhibition of the NO synthesis by FFA also has been reported [35]. Hence, lipotoxicity, glycation of proteins, and oxidative stress may all contribute to the development of the diabetic vasculopathy.

Balancing the cellular responses to lipotoxicity, glucose toxicity, and oxidative stress

The 5′-AMP-activated protein kinase (AMPK) is a serine–threonine kinase that regulates cellular metabolism and function. It was identified originally in the liver where it phosphorylates and inactivates 3-hydroxy-3-methylglutaryl-coenzyme A (CoA) reductase and acetyl-CoA carboxylase (ACC) [39,40]. The physiologic role of AMPK in maintaining cellular energy stores has been deciphered over the past 20 years [41–43]. AMPK is activated when nutrient supply is limited, or ATP generation is impaired, or cellular energy demand is increased. AMPK responds by activating ATP-generating pathways and down-regulating ATP-consuming anabolic pathways. It is now recognized as a "fuel gauge" in mammalian cells and the "guardian of energy status" in the heart [44,45]. AMPK is responsible for the activation of glucose uptake and glycolysis during low-flow ischemia and plays an important protective role in limiting the apoptosis associated with ischemia and reperfusion in the heart. Several human mutations have been described, resulting in cardiac glycogen overload and cardiomyopathy, Wolff-Parkinson-White syndrome, arrhythmias, and heart failure.

The AMPK was first described in 1973 as two different protein kinase activities by two independent observations [39,40]. It was not until 1987 that studies showed that one enzyme was responsible for multiple functions, and it was renamed the AMPK. AMPK exists as a heterotrimer comprising a catalytic α subunit and regulatory β and γ subunits. Each subunit is encoded by multiple genes ($\alpha 1$, $\alpha 2$, $\beta 1$, $\beta 2$, $\gamma 1$, $\gamma 2$, and $\gamma 3$) with splice variants and alternative promoters, thus yielding multiple isoforms. AMP allosterically activates the complex and also promotes activation of AMPK by stimulating phosphorylation of the kinase domain. AMP also inhibits dephosphorylation by protein phosphatases. The fact that AMP activates AMPK by three mechanisms suggests that the system is exquisitely sensitive to small changes in cellular AMP. All three effects of AMP on the AMPK system (allosteric activation, phosphorylation, and inhibition of dephosphorylation) are antagonized by high concentrations of ATP.

The α subunit contains an N-terminal kinase domain and a C-terminal domain involved in complex formation. The β subunits contain conserved C-terminal domains that are sufficient on their own to form a complex with α and γ. The β subunits also contain a carbohydrate-binding domain, the function of which remains unclear, although it has been shown to cause the association of AMPK complexes with glycogen particles, in which one physiologic target (eg, glycogen synthase) resides. In human muscle, there is also evidence that a high cellular glycogen content represses activation of AMPK. This suggests that, in addition to ATP, the AMPK system can also sense its more medium-term availability in the form of glycogen. The γ subunits of AMPK contain four repeats of a sequence motif termed a CBS domain. Each of these domains binds one molecule of AMP or ATP in a mutually exclusive manner, consistent with the findings that high concentrations of ATP antagonize activation of AMPK by AMP. This suggests that isoforms containing certain γ subunits may be more or less sensitive to AMP or ATP and bears further investigation.

From the perspective of lipotoxicity, the activation of AMPK appears to be able to prevent many of the toxic effects. The activation of AMPK increases glucose uptake and glycolysis, diminishes lipid synthesis, and increases the oxidation of fatty acids. The ability to increase oxidation of fatty acids is crucial to prevent lipotoxicity and insulin resistance. However, if AMPK is not inactivated appropriately, it can then contribute to increased ischemic damage in the heart. The heart relies predominantly on a balance between fatty acids and glucose to generate its energy supply. When circulating levels of fatty acids are high, fatty acid oxidation can dominate glucose oxidation as a source of energy. After an ischemic episode, fatty acid oxidation rates increase, resulting in an uncoupling of glycolysis and glucose oxidation. The consequent increase in proton production worsens ischemic damage. Because high rates of fatty acid oxidation also can contribute to ischemic damage by inhibiting glucose oxidation, it is important to maintain the proper control of fatty acid oxidation both during and after ischemia.

An important molecule that controls myocardial fatty acid oxidation is malonyl-CoA, which inhibits the uptake of fatty acids into the mitochondria. The levels of malonyl-CoA in the heart are controlled both by its synthesis and degradation. Three enzymes, namely AMPK, ACC, and malonyl-CoA decarboxylase (MCD), are important in this process. AMPK causes phosphorylation and inhibition of ACC, which reduces the production of malonyl-CoA. AMPK also phosphorylates and activates MCD, promoting the degradation of malonyl-CoA levels. As a result, malonyl-CoA levels can be altered dramatically by the activation of AMPK. In ischemia, AMPK is rapidly activated and inhibits ACC, subsequently decreasing malonyl-CoA levels and increasing fatty acid oxidation rates. The consequence of this reaction is a decrease in glucose oxidation rates. In addition to altering malonyl-CoA levels, AMPK can also increase glycolytic rates, resulting in an increased uncoupling of glycolysis from glucose oxidation and an enhanced production of protons and lactate. If AMPK is not inactivated in a timely manner then this process results in a decrease in cardiac efficiency and contributes to the severity of ischemic damage. There is now a great deal of interest in developing compounds that can alter this system and prevent the progression to heart failure. Therapies to control blood glucose levels must now also target the lipotoxicity and the inflammation and optimize the AMPK system, in addition to lowering glucose to prevent the epidemic of cardiac disease and heart failure that has been developing in recent years.

Glucose-lowering and potential benefits for the heart

Treatment of type 2 diabetes

The currently available classes of antidiabetic agents reduce plasma glucose levels by targeting four processes: (1) the replacement of the relative insufficiency of the pancreatic beta cells either by stimulating the pancreas to produce more insulin (sulfonylureas, nonsulfonylurea secretogogues, and incretin mimetics), by replacing insulin with exogenous insulin, or by replacing amylin deficiency; (2) the stimulation of glucose uptake by muscle and adipose tissues (thiazolidinediones); (3) the reduction of glucose output by the liver (biguanides and thiazolidinediones); and (4) the reduction of glucose absorption by the gut (α-glucosidase inhibitors). However, diet and exercise remain the cornerstones for the management of type 2 diabetes. Caloric restriction, weight loss, and exercise have all been shown to improve vascular and cardiac function in addition to enhancing insulin sensitivity and glycemic control.

Secretogogues

Glucose lowering can be achieved by increasing insulin secretion using secretogogues or by augmenting glucose-stimulated insulin secretion using incretin mimetics. The secretogogues can be separated into two groups: sulfonylureas and nonsulfonylurea secretogogues. A number of sulfonylureas are available because this is one of the oldest classes of antidiabetic agents [46]. The newer or second-generation sulfonylureas (eg, glyburide, glipizide, and glimepiride) are more effective and are associated with lower incidences of adverse events than the older agents are. The nonsulfonylurea secretogogues include two currently available products, nateglinide, a phenylalanine derivative, and repaglinide, a benzoic acid derivative. They have shorter half-lives than sulfonylureas and a reduced risk of hypoglycemia. The secretogogues are useful for lowering glucose but do not have any direct beneficial effects on the heart. In fact, there has been a debate since the University Group Diabetes Program (UGDP) study [47] in the early 1970s regarding the possible deleterious effect of the sulfonylureas since the publication of the university. This study showed an increase in cardiovascular mortality in patients who had type 2 DM taking tolbutamide, a first-generation sulfonylurea [47]. Impaired ischemic preconditioning has been observed in patients taking sulfonylureas, which is likely caused by an effect on the sulfonylurea receptors (SUR). The binding of a sulfonylurea to the cardiac SUR may also block the sarcolemmic K_{ATP} channels, thus impairing cardiac reactivity. For this reason, sulfonylureas would not be the preferred agents in people who have or are at risk for cardiac disease. In addition, the sulfonylureas only lower glucose but do not affect the insulin resistance or inflammation.

Incretin mimetics

The insulin secretory capacity of the pancreatic beta cell also can be augmented by the incretin mimetics. The enhanced insulin response to oral over intravenous glucose is known as the incretin effect. This physiologic observation led to the discovery of compounds now called incretins, such as glucagon-like peptide-1 (GLP-1), produced by the gastrointestinal (GI) tract in response to glucose. GLP-1 and other incretins enhance glucose-dependent insulin secretion and exhibit other antihyperglycemic actions following their release into the circulation from the gut [48]. Synthetic compounds have been developed that have some of the activities of the naturally occurring incretins and have been named "incretin mimetics."

The prototype of this class is exenatide (Byetta), which has been shown to bind and activate the human GLP-1 receptor in vitro [49]. Exenatide mimics certain antihyperglycemic actions of GLP-1, including promoting insulin release from beta cells in the presence of elevated blood glucose concentrations [50]. Exenatide has been shown to augment first- and second-phase insulin secretion in response to intravenous glucose in people who have type 2 DM. Exenatide has been postulated to have effects on organs other than the pancreas but further studies are needed to determine if these effects are clinically relevant.

Amylinomimetics

Pramlintide (Symlin) is a synthetic analog of human amylin, a naturally occurring neuroendocrine hormone synthesized by pancreatic beta cells that contributes to glucose control during the postprandial period. Pramlintide complements the effects of insulin in postprandial glucose regulation by decreasing glucagon secretion. Clinical trials have shown that pramlintide suppresses postmeal glucagon secretion, slows gastric emptying, reduces postprandial glucose levels, and improves glycemic control while managing weight loss [51,52]. Pramlinitide is an injectable agent that is dosed before meals as an adjunct to insulin in patients who have type 1 DM who have not achieved control and in patients who have type 2 DM who use mealtime insulin control [53]. Pramlintide has been associated with an increased risk of insulin-induced severe hypoglycemia; other adverse events include nausea, anorexia, fatigue, and vomiting. Pramlintide has not yet been studied in patients who have kidney failure or heart failure. Pramlintide has been shown to have effects on the GI tract and the brain but has not yet been studied for effects on the heart or vascular system. Pramlintide is not a substitute for insulin and should be used only in combination with insulin.

Thiazolidinediones

The therapeutic benefits of using thiazolidinediones, in addition to glucose lowering, include preservation of beta cell function, augmentation of insulin sensitivity, and minimization of hypoglycemic adverse events [46]. Studies suggest that the thiazolidinediones increase the responsiveness of beta cells by reducing external factors (eg, glucose and free fatty acids) that impair insulin secretion. These same effects of improving the lipotoxicity would also be of benefit to the heart and vascular system. In some systems, these agents have been shown to have beneficial effects on AMPK. This class of agents was approved for use based on their ability to lower glucose; however, they have been shown to improve lipotoxicity, markers of inflammation, and surrogate markers for cardiac risk. A number of outcome studies evaluating the cardiovascular effects of thiazolidinediones are in various stages of completion. The first one to be completed was the Prospective pioglitazone Clinical Trial in Macrovascular Events (PROACTIVE) study by Dormandy and colleagues [16]. PROACTIVE was a double-blinded, placebo-controlled study in which 5238 patients who had type 2 DM and prevalent atherosclerotic vascular disease were randomized to pioglitazone versus placebo. The primary endpoint was a composite of seven major adverse cardiovascular events, including unstable events (all-cause mortality, myocardial infarction [MI], stroke, and acute coronary syndrome) and clinically driven events (coronary or leg revascularization or leg amputation). The study failed to demonstrate a statistically significant difference in the primary endpoint between the treatment groups, with a trend toward a 10% reduction (23.5% versus 21%; $P = .095$) favoring pioglitazone. Treatment with pioglitazone did significantly reduce the principal predefined secondary endpoint, a composite of all-cause mortality-MI-stroke (14.4% versus 12.3%; hazard ratio = 0.84; $P = .027$). These data suggest that the thiazolidinediones do more than just lower glucose and may be of benefit in patients who have diabetes and any amount of vascular disease.

While awaiting the results of the outcome studies, clinicians have had to learn how to deal with the side effects of these agents that have shown promise in treating the deterioration of vascular disease and cardiac function. Thiazolidinediones may cause weight gain and edema when initiated at high doses. The thiazolidinediones have been associated with fluid retention and dilutional anemia, which are caused by an increase in plasma volume and are not recommended for use in patients who have New York Heart Association class 3 or 4 cardiac status because the use of thiazolidinediones in combination with insulin may increase the incidence of cardiac failure [54]. Troglitazone, an older thiazolidinedione, was removed from the market because of hepatotoxicity. Studies show that hepatic failure is not a class effect with these agents; rosiglitazone and pioglitazone have a more favorable hepatic safety profile than troglitazone or placebo.

Biguanides

The primary action of biguanides is to reduce the production of glucose by the liver. Metformin is the only biguanide available in the United States. In the UKPDS study [15], the obese subgroup was randomized to sulfonylurea, insulin, or metformin, and the use of metformin was associated with a decrease in the incidence of myocardial infarction. The mechanism is unknown, but based on these observations, metformin should be used in all patients who do not have a contraindication. Lactic acidosis, a serious metabolic complication, has very rarely been reported with the use of metformin, particularly in individuals who have renal dysfunction or those of advancing age. Serum creatinine levels should be monitored routinely in all patients receiving a biguanide. The US Food and Drug Administration recommends that creatinine clearance be measured before initiating therapy in patients 80 years of age or older [55].

Metformin has been shown to activate AMPK, which would have multiple effects benefiting the heart and endothelium. This may in fact be the mechanism whereby metformin was associated with a decrease in myocardial infarction in the UKPDS. However, the drug is limited to use in the early stages of diabetes because its use is contraindicated in anyone who has renal insufficiency or heart failure.

α-Glucosidase inhibitors

Acarbose and miglitol are α-glucosidase inhibitors that act by delaying carbohydrate absorption in the small intestine. These agents are taken by patients at the beginning of each main meal. The main advantage of the α-glucosidase inhibitors is that they are only minimally absorbed and are rarely associated with hypoglycemia and weight gain. Post hoc analysis of the STOP-NIDDM trial [56] database suggests that the treatment of patients who have IGT with acarbose is associated with a reduction in the risk of cardiovascular disease and hypertension. These data will need to be confirmed in a prospective, randomized, controlled clinical trial. These agents do lower glucose, but it is not yet clear whether they have any beneficial impact on the underlying disease process.

Fixed-dose combinations

Fixed-dose combination pills for the management of type 2 diabetes have been introduced recently in the United States. The advantages include better efficacy with lower doses of each component, improved compliance, increased adherence, fewer complications (eg, less hypoglycemia) caused by lower dosing, and lower expense (the tablets usually are priced at the same cost as the more expensive component alone). The currently available combinations include metformin/glyburide, metformin/glipizide, metformin/rosiglitazone, metformin/pioglitazone, and rosiglitazone/glimepiride. These fixed-dose combination pills allow therapy to be tailored toward treating the underlying disease process of lipotoxicity and insulin resistance in addition to lowering the glucose with the least number of pills.

What about using insulin?

Although insulin has been assumed for many years to have a detrimental effect on the vasculature by virtue of its growth factor-like effect, recent data have shown that insulin exerts desirable actions on the vasculature, primarily by amplifying endothelium-dependent vasodilation, increasing endothelial constitutive nitric oxide synthase gene expression and activity and, therefore, NO bioavailability, which in turn exerts a wide array of antiatherogenic actions [57]. Consequently, insulin resistance in the endothelial cell decreases or prevents these beneficial actions of insulin [34,58]. The inappropriate elevation of plasma FFAs seen in insulin resistance is associated with a decrease in circulating levels of most amino acids, including L-arginine, which may reduce the substrate for NO formation. Given the relationship between endothelial dysfunction and atherosclerosis, it is likely that the status of endothelial function may reflect the propensity of an individual to develop atherosclerotic disease. Consequently, the beneficial effect of insulin on decreasing endothelial activation, thereby improving endothelial dysfunction, raises the possibility that insulin therapy should be initiated much earlier in the disease process than it has been under traditional diabetes management.

Summary

Diabetes is a multiorgan disease. Therapy must now be targeted toward treating the underlying disease process and not just lowering the serum glucose level. Preventing the vascular disease and progression to heart failure has become an important goal of therapy as the epidemic of obesity and type 2 diabetes explodes. Heart failure is no longer limited to the geriatric population. With type 2 DM now being identified in youth and adolescents, heart failure will soon be seen in people in their third and fourth decades. Therapies to control blood glucose must now target the lipotoxicity and the inflammation and optimize the AMPK system, in addition to lowering glucose, to prevent the epidemic of cardiac disease and heart failure that has been developing in recent years.

References

[1] Kannel W, McGee D. Diabetes and cardiovascular disease: the Framingham Study. JAMA 1979;241(19): 2035–8.

[2] Kannel W, McGee D. Diabetes and glucose tolerance as risk factors for cardiovascular disease: the Framingham Study. Diabetes Care 1979;2(2):120–6.

[3] Pyörälä K, Laakso M, Uusitupa M. Diabetes and atherosclerosis: an epidemiologic view. Diabetes Metab Rev 1987;3(2):463–524.

[4] Bierman E. George Lyman Duff Memorial Lecture: atherogenesis in diabetes. Arterioscler Thromb 1992; 12(6):647–56.

[5] Butler W, Ostrander Jr L, Carman W, et al. Mortality from coronary heart disease in the Tecumseh study: long-term effect of diabetes mellitus, glucose tolerance and other risk factors. Am J Epidemiol 1985;121(4): 541–7.

[6] Klein R. Hyperglycemia and microvascular and macrovascular disease in diabetes. Diabetes Care 1995;18(2): 258–68.

[7] Kleinman J, Donahue R, Harris M, et al. Mortality among diabetics in a national sample. Am J Epidemiol 1988;128(2):389–401.

[8] Kuller LH, Velentgas P, Barzilay J, et al. Diabetes mellitus: subclinical cardiovascular disease and risk of incident cardiovascular disease and all-cause mortality. Arterioscler Thromb Vasc Biol 2000;20(3):823–9.

[9] Olson J, Edmundowicz D, Becker D, et al. Coronary calcium in adults with type 1 diabetes: a stronger correlate of clinical coronary artery disease in men than in women. Diabetes 2000;49(9):1571–8.

[10] Lloyd CE, Kuller LH, Ellis D, et al. Coronary artery disease in IDDM: gender differences in risk factors but not risk. Arterioscler Thromb Vasc Biol 1996; 16(6):720–6.

[11] Barzilay JI, Spiekerman CF, Kuller LH, et al. Prevalence of clinical and isolated subclinical cardiovascular disease in older adults with glucose disorders: the Cardiovascular Health Study. Diabetes Care 2001; 24(7):1233–9.

[12] The DECODE Study Group on behalf of the European Diabetes Epidemiology Group. Age, body mass index and glucose tolerance in 11 European population-based surveys. Diabet Med 2002;19(7):558–65.

[13] The Diabetes Control and Complications Trial Research Group. The effect of intensive treatment of diabetes on the development and progression of long-term complications in insulin-dependent diabetes mellitus. N Engl J Med 1993;329(14):977–86.

[14] UK Prospective Diabetes Study (UKPDS) Group. Intensive blood-glucose control with sulphonylureas or insulin compared with conventional treatment and

risk of complications in patients with type 2 diabetes (UKPDS 33). Lancet 1998;352(9131):837–53.

[15] UK Prospective Diabetes Study (UKPDS) Group. Effect of intensive blood-glucose control with metformin on complications in overweight patients with type 2 diabetes (UKPDS 34). Lancet 1998;352(9131): 854–65.

[16] Dormandy JA, Charbonnel B, Eckland DJ, et al. Secondary prevention of macrovascular events in patients with type 2 diabetes in the PROactive Study (PROspective pioglitAzone Clinical Trial In macroVascular Events): a randomised controlled trial. Lancet 2005; 366(9493):1279–89.

[17] The Diabetes Control and Complications Trial/Epidemiology of Diabetes Interventions and Complications (DCCT/EDIC) Study Research Group. Intensive diabetes treatment and cardiovascular disease in patients with type 1 diabetes. N Engl J Med 2005;353(25): 2643–53.

[18] Shichiri M, Kishikawa H, Ohkubo Y, et al. Long-term results of the Kumamoto Study on optimal diabetes control in type 2 diabetic patients. Diabetes Care 2000; 23(Suppl 2):B21.

[19] Unger RH, Orci L. Lipoapoptosis: its mechanism and its diseases. Biochim Biophys Acta 2002;1585(2–3): 202–12.

[20] Tomas E, Kelly M, Xiang X, et al. Metabolic and hormonal interactions between muscle and adipose tissue. Proc Nutr Soc 2004;63(2):381–5.

[21] Unger RH. Lipid overload and overflow: metabolic trauma and the metabolic syndrome. Trends Endocrinol Metab 2003;14(9):398–403.

[22] Hotamisligil GS. Role of endoplasmic reticulum stress and c-Jun NH2-terminal kinase pathways in inflammation and origin of obesity and diabetes. Diabetes 2005;54(Suppl 2):S73–8.

[23] Wellen KE, Hotamisligil GS. Obesity-induced inflammatory changes in adipose tissue. J Clin Invest 2003; 112(12):1785–8.

[24] Costacou T, Zgibor JC, Evans RW, et al for the Pittsburgh Epidemiology of Diabetes Complications Study. The prospective association between adiponectin and coronary artery disease among individuals with type 1 diabetes. Diabetologia 2005;48(1):41–8.

[25] Orchard TJ, Olson JC, Erbey JR, et al. Insulin resistance-related factors, but not glycemia, predict coronary artery disease in type 1 diabetes: 10-year follow-up data from the Pittsburgh Epidemiology of Diabetes Complications study. Diabetes Care 2003; 26(5):1374–9.

[26] Brownlee M, Vassara H, Cerami A. Nonenzymatic glycosylation and the pathogenesis of diabetes complications. Ann Intern Med 1984;101:527–37.

[27] Nishikawa T, Edelstein D, Brownlee M. The missing link: a single unifying mechanism for diabetic complications. KI 2000;58(77):S26–30.

[28] Schmidt AM, Yan SD, Wautier JL, et al. Activation of receptor for advanced glycation end products: a mechanism for chronic vascular dysfunction in diabetic

vasculopathy and atherosclerosis. Circ Res 1999;84(5): 489–97.

[29] Wendt T, Harja E, Bucciarelli L, et al. RAGE modulates vascular inflammation and atherosclerosis in a murine model of type 2 diabetes. Atherosclerosis 2006; 185(1):70–7.

[30] Koyama H, Shoji T, Yokoyama H, et al. Plasma level of endogenous secretory rage is associated with components of the metabolic syndrome and atherosclerosis. Arterioscler Thromb Vasc Biol 2005;25(12):2587–93.

[31] Koivisto V, Stevens L, Mattock M, et al for the EURODIAB IDDM Complications Study Group. Cardiovascular disease and its risk factors in IDDM in Europe. Diabetes Care 1996;19(7):689–97.

[32] Orchard T, Stevens L, Forrest K, et al. Cardiovascular disease in insulin dependent diabetes mellitus: similar rates but different risk factors in the US compared with Europe. Int J Epidemiol 1998;27(6):976–83.

[33] Cai H, Harrison DG. Endothelial dysfunction in cardiovascular diseases: the role of oxidant stress. Circ Res 2000;87(10):840–4.

[34] Steinberg HO, Chaker H, Leaming R, et al. Obesity/insulin resistance is associated with endothelial dysfunction. implications for the syndrome of insulin resistance. J Clin Invest 1996;97(11):2601–10.

[35] Davda RK, Stepniakowski KT, Lu G, et al. Oleic acid inhibits endothelial nitric oxide synthase by a protein kinase C-independent mechanism. Hypertension 1995; 26(5):764–70.

[36] Giugliano D, Ceriello A, Paolisso G. Diabetes mellitus, hypertension, and cardiovascular disease: which role for oxidative stress? Metabolism 1995;44(3):363–8.

[37] Pleiner J, Schaller G, Mittermayer F, et al. FFA-induced endothelial dysfunction can be corrected by vitamin C. J Clin Endocrinol Metab 2002;87(6): 2913–7.

[38] Ferrannini E, Barrett EJ, Bevilacqua S, et al. Effect of free fatty acids on blood amino acid levels in human. Am J Physiol Endocrinol Metab 1986;250(6):E686–94.

[39] Beg Z, Allmann D, Gibson D. Modulation of 3-hydroxy-3-methylglutaryl coenzyme A reductase activity with cAMP and with protein fractions of rat liver cytosol. Biochem Biophys Res Commun 1973; 54(4):1362–9.

[40] Carlson C, Kim K. Regulation of hepatic acetyl coenzyme A carboxylase by phosphorylation and dephosphorylation. J Biol Chem 1973;248(1):378–80.

[41] Carling D, Zammit V, Hardie D. A common bicyclic protein kinase cascade inactivates the regulatory enzymes of fatty acid and cholesterol biosynthesis. FEBS Lett 1987;223(2):217–22.

[42] Sim A, Hardie D. The low activity of acetyl-CoA carboxylase in basal and glucagon-stimulated hepatocytes is due to phosphorylation by the AMPactivated protein kinase kinase and not cyclic AMP-dependent protein kinase. FEBS Lett 1988;233:294–8.

[43] Hardie D, Carling D, The ATRS. AMP-activated protein kinase—a multisubstrate regulator of lipid metabolism. Trends Biochem Sci 1989;14:20–3.

[44] Hardie D, Carling D. The AMP-activated protein kinase-fuel gauge of the mammalian cell? Eur J Biochem 1997;246:259–73.

[45] Hardie D. AMP-activated protein kinase: the guardian of cardiac energy status. J Clin Invest 2004;114: 465–8.

[46] Inzucchi SE. Oral antihyperglycemic therapy for type 2 diabetes: scientific review. JAMA 2002;287(3):360–72.

[47] Meinert C, Knatterud G, Prout T, et al. A study of the effects of hypoglycemic agents on vascular complications in patients with adult-onset diabetes: II. mortality results. Diabetes 1970;19(Suppl):S789–830.

[48] D'Alessio DA, Vahl TP. Glucagon-like peptide 1: evolution of an incretin into a treatment for diabetes. Am J Physiol Endocrinol Metab 2004;286(6):E882–90.

[49] Koyama H, Shoji T, Yokoyama H, et al. Plasma level of endogenous secretory rage is associated with components of the metabolic syndrome and atherosclerosis. Arterioscler Thromb Vasc Biol 2005;25(12):2587–93.

[50] Kolterman OG, Kim DD, Shen L, et al. Pharmacokinetics, pharmacodynamics, and safety of exenatide in patients with type 2 diabetes mellitus. Am J Health Syst Pharm 2005;62(2):173–81.

[51] Chapman I, Parker B, Doran S, et al. Effect of pramlintide on satiety and food intake in obese subjects and subjects with type 2 diabetes. Diabetologia 2005; 48(5):838–48.

[52] Ceriello A, Piconi L, Quagliaro L, et al. Effects of pramlintide on postprandial glucose excursions and measures of oxidative stress in patients with type 1 diabetes. Diabetes Care 2005;28(3):632–7.

[53] Yonekura H, Yamamoto Y, Sakurai S, et al. Roles of the receptor for advanced glycation end products in diabetes-induced vascular injury. J Pharmacol Sci 2005;97(3):305–11.

[54] Nesto RW, Bell D, Bonow RO, et al. Thiazolidinedione use, fluid retention, and congestive heart failure: a consensus statement from the American Heart Association and American Diabetes Association. Diabetes Care 2004;27(1):256–63.

[55] Bristol-Myers Squibb Company. Glucophage/Glucophage XR [package insert: prescribing information]. Princeton (NJ): Bristol-Myers Squibb Company; 2004.

[56] Chiasson J-L, Josse RG, Gomis R, et al. Acarbose treatment and the risk of cardiovascular disease and hypertension in patients with impaired glucose tolerance: the STOP-NIDDM Trial. JAMA 2003;290(4): 486–94.

[57] Hotamisligil GS. Inflammatory pathways and insulin action. Int J Obes Relat Metab Disord 2003; 27(Suppl 3):S53–5.

[58] Arcaro G, Cretti A, Balzano S, et al. Insulin causes endothelial dysfunction in humans: sites and mechanisms. Circulation 2002;105(5):576–82.

ELSEVIER
SAUNDERS

Heart Failure Clin 2 (2006) 71 – 80

HEART
FAILURE
CLINICS

Diabetic Cardiomyopathy

T. Brooks Vaughan, MD[a],*, David S.H. Bell, MB, FRCPEd, FRCPC[b]

[a]University of Alabama at Birmingham, Birmingham, AL, USA
[b]Private Practice, Birmingham, AL, USA

Congestive heart failure (CHF) is commonly associated with diabetes. In years past, it was assumed that this association was largely based on the increased risk in the diabetic patient for ischemic heart disease. More recently, it has become evident that the relationship between these two diseases is more complex than was originally thought. The concept of a diabetic cardiomyopathy, independent of other known causes of cardiomyopathy (ischemic, hypertensive, alcoholic, or viral) has emerged as a potential explanation for this relationship. This article assesses the epidemiologic relationship between diabetes and cardiomyopathy and several major avenues of investigation into its pathophysiology.

Epidemiology

As early as 1979, the Framingham Heart Study demonstrated that heart failure (HF) was twice as common in diabetic men and five times as common in diabetic women aged 45 to 75 years as in age-matched control subjects. This association grew stronger in younger patients (<65 years), being fourfold higher in diabetic male patients and eightfold higher in diabetic female patients than in nondiabetic subjects

[1]. A more recent health maintenance organization study of nearly 10,000 patients with type II diabetes demonstrated that 12% of subjects had HF at entry and that risk factors for HF were greater age, longer duration of diabetes, use of insulin, and lower body mass index (BMI). The more than 8000 patients who did not have HF at entry went on to develop HF at the alarming rate of 3.3% per year [2].

A study of nursing home residents initially free of HF revealed that 39% of those who had diabetes and 23% of those who did not have diabetes had developed HF after 43 months of follow-up, a relative risk (RR) of 1.3 [3]. A cross-sectional Italian study found the prevalence of diabetes to be 30% in an elderly HF population [4]. Another Italian study investigated the predictors of death from HF in an elderly population initially free of HF at enrollment. Diabetes was actually a stronger predictor of death than a clinical history of coronary artery disease (RR 1.35 versus 1.25) [5].

The economic impact of this association is significant. Patients who have diabetes account for more than 33% of all patients requiring hospitalization for HF, and the actual number may approach 50% [6,7]. In Alabama in 2000, the diagnosis of diabetes accompanied 38% of patients admitted to a tertiary care hospital, a rate similar to the 33.6% found in a statewide quality assurance audit [8]. In large-scale clinical trials, the prevalence of diabetes is high but is somewhat lower than in studies of hospital admissions. This finding may represent selection bias against patients with coexistent renal insufficiency. Nonetheless, diabetic patients represented approximately 25% of those outpatients enrolled in Studies of Left Ventricular Dysfunction (SOLVD), Meto-

* Corresponding author. Division of Diabetes, Endocrinology, and Metabolism, University of Alabama at Birmingham, 510 20th Street South, Suite 702, FOT, Birmingham, AL 35294.
E-mail address: brooks@uab.edu (T.B. Vaughan).

1551-7136/06/$ – see front matter © 2006 Elsevier Inc. All rights reserved.
doi:10.1016/j.hfc.2005.11.001

heartfailure.theclinics.com

prolol Controlled-Release Randomized Intervention Trial in Heart Failure, and Evaluation of Losartan in the Elderly trials. The prevalence of diabetes in hospitalized patients with CHF was even higher, representing 44% and 47%, respectively, of patients in Outcomes of a Prospective Trial of Intravenous Milrinone for Exacerbations of Chronic Heart Failure and Vasodilation in the Management of Acute CHF [7].

Interestingly, HF may represent an independent risk factor for the development of diabetes. During a 3-year follow-up of nondiabetic HF patients, diabetes developed in 29%, compared with 18% of matched control subjects. Multivariate analysis supported HF as being a risk factor for diabetes [4]. This relationship has been suggested in other studies as well, with multiple factors being implicated, including decreased physical activity in these patients due to symptomatology. Another possible factor is the pro-inflammatory and hyperadrenergic state induced by HF, which may lead to insulin resistance [9,10].

An independent association

First reported in 1972, epidemiologic evidence that a disease-specific cardiomyopathy may exist in the diabetic patient has been suggestive, but the data are clouded by the multiple causes of CHF [11]. A lack of uniformity in diagnostic criteria has also made this a challenging entity to study. Previous studies associating diabetes and CHF have excluded ischemic cardiomyopathy and some other potential causes, but their criteria have varied [12]. A large case-control study was recently conducted in an attempt to account for more of the potential confounding diagnoses. The authors used the 1995 Nationwide Inpatient Sample, which includes more than 900 hospitals in 19 states. They evaluated patients who were discharged with a diagnosis of idiopathic cardiomyopathy (ICM), defined as a primary cardiomyopathy without the following comorbidities: pregnancy, ischemic heart disease, valvular heart disease, alcoholism, thyroid disease, HIV infection or AIDS, amyloidosis, myocarditis, and chemotherapy-related diagnoses [13]. They found a relative odds ratio of receiving a diagnosis of ICM in the diabetic patient of 1.75 (95% confidence interval 1.71–1.79). More alarmingly, the authors found a discharge rate for ICM of 7.6 per 1000 in patients who had diabetes. As the authors point out, this approaches the discharge rate for diabetes-related lower-extremity amputation (9.4 per 1000) [13].

Echocardiographic evidence

Much of the above-mentioned epidemiologic evidence correlating diabetes and cardiomyopathy involves patients with clinically evident systolic dysfunction. Using sophisticated ultrasound techniques, one finds that diabetic cardiomyopathy is present in a preclinical state far earlier than might be appreciated by even the most skilled examiner. These early abnormalities have repeatedly been demonstrated using Doppler ultrasound techniques. Tissue Doppler (which actually looks at tissue, usually the mitral annulus, rather than blood flow) appears to represent a less pre-load dependent and more linear expression of diastolic dysfunction than do more traditional echocardiographic methods [14]. The earliest manifestations are generally evident in measures of diastolic function. Evidence of diastolic dysfunction, characterized by impairment in early diastolic filling, prolongation of isovolumetric relaxation, increased atrial filling, and increased ventricular wall dimension, has been shown even in young patients with type I diabetes [15]. A recent study of 80 children and adolescents with type I diabetes and matched controls using echocardiography, including tissue Doppler techniques, showed evidence of left ventricular structural and filling abnormalities, with more pronounced findings in girls than in boys [16]. This finding is notable, considering that adult studies, including the Framingham Heart Study, suggest stronger risks versus their nondiabetic peers (5.1 fold) for CHF in women than in men (2.4 fold) [1].

As ultrasound techniques improve, the prevalence of diabetic cardiomyopathy appears to be increasing. Studies conducted in the 1990s showed a prevalence of diastolic dysfunction in the range of 30% [17,18]. More recent studies using Doppler techniques have accounted for pseudonormalization (which may have confounded earlier data) and have shown an even higher prevalence of abnormalities. The prevalence of diastolic dysfunction in diabetic patients in Olmstead County, Minnesota was 52% [19]. Poirier and colleagues [20] showed a prevalence of diastolic dysfunction of 60% in well-controlled type II diabetic patients.

Early evidence of systolic dysfunction has been noted as well, both in children who have diabetes and in adults [21,22]. Again, more sophisticated ultrasound techniques will most likely elucidate subtle abnormalities in systolic dysfunction. Fang and colleagues [23] recently published a study of 186 patients who had normal ejection fractions and no evidence of coronary artery disease and were able to discern differences in systolic function between diabetic patients and controls by measuring parameters such as peak strain and strain rate.

Causation

Advanced glycosylation end products

Although epidemiologic studies specifically addressing diabetic cardiomyopathy are limited, physiologic evidence indicates its existence. Multiple lines of evidence suggest various pathophysiologic mechanisms. Certain aspects of diabetic cardiomyopathy are shared by those with type I and type II diabetes, despite their different metabolic defects. This evidence suggests that hyperglycemia could be a unifying mechanism. In fact, most (though not all) studies support an association between glycemic control and worsening cardiomyopathy [24,25]. In the Strong Heart Study, the extent and frequency of diastolic dysfunction was directly proportional to the hemoglobin A1c level [26]. A potential explanation is the formation of advanced glycosylation end products (AGE) in the myocardium. In animal studies, the presence of diabetes results in increased myocardial AGE receptor expression, increased cross-linking of collagen, and myocardial fibrosis [27]. With lysis of collagen cross-links in animal models, there was a decrease in myocardial fibrosis and an improvement in diastolic function [28]. Rats with demonstrated formation of AGE who were treated with alagebrium chloride (a cross-link breaker) showed reduced left ventricular mass and reduced expression of brain natriuretic peptide [27]. The existence of fibrosis in diabetic patients is supported by biopsy studies as well as by newer, less invasive strategies [29]. Ultrasonic backscatter has been shown to correlate with the degree of collagen deposition [30], and Fang and colleagues [23] have noted an increase in myocardial reflectivity by ultrasound in diabetic patients without known coronary artery disease versus controls.

Another potential noninvasive marker of fibrosis is procollagen type I c-peptide, which has still to be validated in large, long-term trials. Some evidence currently links it with collagen production and CHF [31]. Gonzalez-Vilchez and colleagues [31] were able to demonstrate a correlation between preclinical echocardiographic abnormalities and serum levels of procollagen type I c-peptide in patients who had type II diabetes and no known cardiac disease.

Although these findings represent a significant possible source of pathology as well as an oppor-tunity for intervention in diabetic cardiomyopathy, it appears likely that other mechanisms are at work. This notion is supported by two studies of children who had diabetes in which a correlation between duration of diabetes, hemoglobin A1c, and preclinical echocardiographic dysfunction was not established [16]. In addition, epidemiologic data support improved glycemic control as a way to lessen the risk of death or hospitalization from CHF [24]. Physiologic support for this hypothesis is provided by studies that show improvement in echocardiographic parameters (backscatter, diastolic and systolic function) and a certain degree of pathologic change in response to improved glycemic control [25]. The formation of AGE is an irreversible process; in the absence of collagen, lysis would not be expected to vanish with improved glycemic control [27].

Metabolic defects

The metabolic effects of hyperglycemia and glycation may explain the relationship of cardiomyopathy to glycemic control. Glycation and glycoxidation by free radicals of the sarcolemmal membrane alter calcium homeostasis, leading to calcium resistance in diabetic hearts. This resistance in turn leads to myocardial dysfunction, which may be reversed with an aminoguanidine-induced reduction in glycosylation [32]. This effect has been illustrated in rats by evidence of a reduction in fructosamines (a glycation end-product) in sarcolemmal membranes with these agents. Additionally, aminoguanidines appear to have another beneficial effect in terms of "fluidizing" the membrane lipid bilayer and lessening calcium resistance. Our understanding of this process is incomplete, because this calcium resistance may be protective against metabolic disturbances; there is some evidence that reversing this process in the setting of hyperglycemia may be maladaptive, as discussed later in this article [32].

Hyperglycemia also increases the myocardial content of free radicals and oxidants, a process that decreases nitric oxide levels, causes DNA damage, worsens endothelial function, and induces myocardial inflammation through stimulation of poly−(ADP-ribose) polymerase−1 (PARP). Evidence for this effects exists in both murine and human endothelial cells [33]. It has been shown that this loss of endothelial function is reversible with PARP inhibition [34]. It is speculated that PARP inhibition prevents upregulation of the proinflammatory pathways that are triggered by hyperglycemia and conserves cellular energetic pools by means of preservation of NADPH [34].

Lipotoxicity due to the elevation of free fatty acids (FFAs) associated with hyperglycemia or insulin resistance almost certainly plays some role in diabetic cardiomyopathy. FFAs are thought to have a variety of direct toxic effects, including disruption of the plasma membrane and alteration of calcium metabolism [35,36]. Excess FFAs most likely accumulate in the diabetic heart (a hypothesis supported by rat studies) and induce activation of the nuclear receptor PPARα [37,38]. Induction of PPARα, both pharmacologically and by gene overexpression, has been shown in animal models to induce cardiac dysfunction and a pattern of metabolism similar to that of the diabetic heart [38,39].

Copper metabolism is another promising area of recent study. Cooper and colleagues [40] have recently demonstrated that treatment with trientine, a copper selective chelating agent, improves cardiac structure in rats and mitigates left ventricular hypertrophy (LVH) in humans. They have also demonstrated that diabetic humans have a tendency toward positive copper balance and speculate that build-up of copper in the extracellular matrix leads to free radical formation [41]. The build-up may be driven by hyperglycemia, which may have inhibitory effects on the copper-binding capacity of ceruloplasmin and albumin. The authors' hypothesis is supported by evidence of correlation between levels of extracellular superoxide dismutase (a potential marker of vascular injury) and serum copper levels in diabetic subjects, as well as by suppression of extracellular superoxide dismutase activity with chelation therapy [41].

Activation of fetal gene program

In animal studies, activation of protein kinase C (PKC)–B activity by hyperglycemia has resulted in myocardial necrosis and fibrosis and ventricular dysfunction (independent of vascular dysfunction). The administration to rats of an oral inhibitor of PKC-B resulted in both functional and histologic improvement [42].

The activation of PKC may play a role, along with activation of the renin-angiotensin system and sympathetic nervous system, in the alteration of gene expression to what has been called the fetal gene program. Atrial natriuretic peptide, which is ordinarily limited to atrial muscle, is re-expressed in the ventricle, as it was in fetal life. The proportions of the fast (α) and slow (β) isoforms of myosin heavy chain (MHC) are changed to a more fetal-like pattern, with higher β-MHC and lower α-MHC. The skeletal muscle α actin gene, which is not expressed in

cardiac muscle after birth, is also re-expressed in the heart along with the normal cardiac actin gene. As these genes are being re-expressed, there is downregulation of the gene encoding a key ionotropic protein, sarcoplasmic reticular Ca ATPase. The net effect may serve as an adaptive mechanism to the surviving myocardium by reducing its energy expenditure [43,44].

Microvascular disease

Although coronary artery disease is associated with diabetes, it is not uncommon for the diabetic patient to have HF in the absence of coronary artery disease. Thus, the presence of microvascular disease is a proposed mechanism for diabetic cardiomyopathy.

In general, microvascular ischemia has been excluded by the absence of increased lactate production during atrial pacing in such patients and by biopsy studies showing no differences between intramyocardial vessels of diabetic subjects and those of controls with cardiomyopathy [45,46].

Defective angiogenesis in response to hypoxia has been reported in diabetic patients, and this could lead to a decrease in capillary density and an ischemic cardiomyopathy [47]. Vascular endothelial growth factor (VEGF) is a promoter of hypoxia-induced neovascularization. It is known that mice lacking VEGF develop severe cardiomyopathy and that VEGF is downregulated in human cardiomyopathy. Yoon and colleagues [48] originally demonstrated a downregulation of VEGF expression in diabetic mice after hindlimb ischemia, but more recently they demonstrated downregulation in diabetic rats without the intentional induction of physiologic stress. VEGF downregulation preceded the development of diabetic cardiomyopathy, and improvements in both function and structure followed the restoration of VEGF expression by intramyocardial gene transfer of plasmid DNA encoding human VEGF. As the authors point out, this model was in streptozotocin-induced diabetic rats, and the metabolic milieu does not mimic type II diabetes.

Autonomic dysfunction

The presence of cardiovascular autonomic neuropathy probably contributes to diabetic cardiomyopathy as well. The mechanisms of diabetic neuropathy are themselves a topic of some controversy, with metabolic, neurohormonal, and autoimmune factors potentially at work, as well as neurovascular insufficiency [49]. The prevalence of cardiovascular autonomic neuropathy (CAN) is unclear, with estimates ranging from 7% to 90% in diabetic patients [49]. Difficulties in standardizing degree of glycemic control, duration of diabetes, and definition of CAN account for some of this variability. The primary manifestations of CAN include diminishment of heart rate variability, resting tachycardia (and potentially bradycardia), orthostatic hypotension, and the potential for silent myocardial ischemia [49,50]. Some consensus exists that CAN is first manifested in reduced heart rate variability [49,50]. The presence of CAN portends a fivefold elevation in 5-year mortality, a potentially increased risk of arrhythmia, a two- to threefold elevation in operative mortality, and a diminished quality of life [50].

Vinik and colleagues [49] recently reviewed the potential causes of elevated mortality in the diabetic patient with CAN. A link to cardiovascular mortality is clearly established, as is a link to left ventricular dysfunction [49–51]. Potential mechanisms include an impaired respiratory response to hypoxia, impaired potential to recognize hypoglycemia, acceleration of microvascular complications, and perturbation of circadian sympathetic and blood pressure variation [49]. More direct lines of evidence are emerging. These include studies with meta-iodobenzylguanidine (^{123}I-MiBG) showing diminished uptake in individuals with CAN, implying cardiac sympathetic dysfunction, and other studies showing diminished cardiac perfusion compared with controls [52,53].

Sympathetic and renin-angiotensin activation

Experimental models of diabetic cardiomyopathy show the same biochemical and molecular abnormalities in the myocardium that occur with hemodynamic overload, offering a common pathway for treatment. Hyperglycemia alone has been shown to activate the same pathways (PKC and mitogen-activated protein kinase) that are activated by hemodynamic overload in mechanical stretch or increased ventricular wall stress [54]. Activation of these pathways leads to decreased myocardial performance, which leads to activation of the renin-angiotensin system (RAS) and the sympathetic nervous system (SNS) to avoid hypoperfusion.

Although initially protective, persistent stimulation of the RAS and SNS and other autocrine and paracrine systems leads to progressive loss of cardiac myocytes. This effect is due to accelerated myocardial apoptosis and necrosis, which in turn lead to further myocardial dysfunction and the downward spiral of cardiac failure. In addition, activation of the RAS and SNS causes cellular hypertrophy and changes in the size and shape of the left ventricle (remodeling). Although remodeling results in an increase in myocardial mass, the placement of the muscle is such that it worsens rather than improves myocardial performance.

This deterioration in myocardial function further stimulates the RAS and SNS, resulting in an acceleration of the remodeling process and further deterioration in myocardial function. Eventually, myocardial function declines to a level that results in HF. Thus, a process that initially is adaptive and protective eventually results in compromised myocardial function and HF [55].

Diagnosis

Risk factors

Clinically, diabetic cardiomyopathy is indistinguishable from any other form of HF in the diabetic patient. The high prevalence and significant morbidity and mortality of HF mandate early identification of risk factors and clinical signs so that one may deliver appropriate and timely therapy. Although treatment has been shown to reduce the complications of HF, approximately 50% of individuals who have left ventricular systolic dysfunction—the antecedent to HF—remain undiagnosed and untreated [56]. Early diagnosis and immediate treatment may help delay or prevent the progression of this debilitating disease.

Risk factor identification may be the most reliable indicator of subclinical myocardial dysfunction. The most prominent risk factors for HF in both diabetic and nondiabetic individuals include prior myocardial infarction (especially anterior or Q-wave), angina pectoris, hypertension, and valvular deformity [57,58]. Diabetes has such an important influence on the development of HF that it has been incorporated as a risk factor in the American College of Cardiology/American Heart Association HF guidelines [59]. In the Sixth Report of the Joint National Committee on Prevention, Detection, Evaluation, and Treatment of High Blood Pressure, the guidelines place patients who have diabetes automatically in the highest risk category for HF, even with high-normal blood pressure and no target organ damage [60]. Increased age, longer duration of diabetes, use of insulin, and increased body weight independently contribute to the risk for HF [24]. The macrovascular and microvascular risks associated with type II diabetes are strongly associated with an increased blood pressure [61].

Screening

A careful history will detect symptoms of dyspnea on effort, orthopnea, nocturnal cough or wheezing, easy fatigability, and nocturia. However, as discussed by Marantz and colleagues [62], many patients who have left ventricular systolic dysfunction do not report symptoms (eg, 20% of those with an ejection fraction <40%). In many cases, this lack of symptoms may be due to absolute inactivity; a simple in-office exercise tolerance examination can be revealing. Time to dyspnea may be judged by simply walking the patient or observing the patient on a graded exercise test [63].

Physical examination may not show signs of HF, no matter how skilled the examiner. In the SOLVD study, among those subjects with an ejection fraction of less than 45%, 32% were observed to have rales, 26% to have edema, 26% to have jugular vein distention, and 17% to have a third heart sound [64]. Therefore, the diagnosis of HF in the diabetic patient may require further testing. Although electrocardiogram and chest radiography may be helpful in demonstrating hypertrophy, which is present in 32% of diabetic patients, or left ventricular enlargement, two-dimensional and pulsed Doppler echocardiography is needed to visualize the cardiac structural and functional changes that underlie HF. This is the recommended test when HF is suspected [65,66]. An economical test to prescreen patients for left ventricular dysfunction and the need for echocardiographic evaluation is the plasma level of brain natriuretic peptide (BNP). Like atrial natriuretic peptide (ANP), BNP is elevated with increased cardiac filling pressure, but unlike ANP, it is not affected by hyperglycemia [67]. Used as a screening test in patients aged more than 55 years, BNP had a sensitivity of 92% and a specificity of 72% [68]. Therefore, plasma BNP level may be an excellent and economical test for identifying diabetic patients who should be further evaluated for HF with echocardiography.

Another test of left ventricular dysfunction, which should be performed in all diabetic patients on a yearly basis, is analysis of urine for microalbuminuria. The Strong Heart Study showed that the degree of diastolic dysfunction was proportional to the level of microalbuminuria, even after adjusting for age, sex, BMI, systolic blood pressure, duration of diabetes, left ventricular mass, and presence of coronary artery disease [69]. Furthermore, the Heart Outcomes Prevention Evaluation study showed that the presence of microalbuminuria was associated with significant risk for CHF [70]. Because microalbuminuria is a marker of endothelial dysfunction in the glomerulus, which is an arteriole, it is logical to postulate that endothelial dysfunction in the myocardium leads to increased ventricular scarring and stiffness, due to either reperfusion injury or exudation of protein from the vessel wall. Therefore, the presence or development of microalbuminuria warrants the cost of echocardiography with pulsed-wave Doppler evaluation, even in the asymptomatic diabetic patient.

Treatment

The ideal treatment for diabetic cardiomyopathy is prevention. Although we lack prospective epidemiologic data regarding diabetic cardiomyopathy in particular, we may draw some conclusions based on our knowledge of established risk factors for HF and on strong pathophysiologic data. Clearly, meticulous control of blood pressure, hyperlipidemia, and glycemia in the diabetic patient should be maintained. Over large populations, an association between increasing hemoglobin A1c and increased risk of HF is clearly established, and the United Kingdom Prospective Diabetes Study demonstrated a reduction in HF as blood pressure control improved [71,72].

In terms of medical therapy, established therapies that alter the maladaptive response to HF, such as β-blockade and RAS blockade, should be employed. These drugs address mechanisms at work in all forms of CHF. In terms of diabetic cardiomyopathy in particular, both metformin and the thiazolidinediones represent potential therapies, although their use in the setting of CHF is controversial because of concerns about lactic acidosis and fluid retention, respectively.

Although metformin does act as an insulin sensitizer, this is not its primary mechanism of action. Thiazolidinediones (Peroxisome proliferator activated receptors [PPAR]-γ agonists) have been demonstrated to improve both whole-body and cardiac insulin sensitivity along with other cardiovascular parameters [73]. Current evidence suggests that thiazolidinedione-associated fluid retention is actually more likely to manifest in terms of peripheral edema than pulmonary edema, elevated central venous pressure, or ascites, even in the setting of class I or II HF [8]. No detriment to cardiac function has been demonstrated in the setting of thiazolidinedione use [74–76]. Further trials of the use of thiazolidinediones in HF are ongoing.

A large observational study recently evaluated readmission rates and mortality in more than 16,000 Medicare patients discharged from the hospital with the diagnoses of diabetes and HF [77]. The investigators compared outcomes for those patients given metformin, thiazolidinediones, and neither drug. A statistically significant improvement in mortality at 1 year was seen in both the metformin and thiazolidinedione groups compared with the group on neither drug. Readmission rates for HF were slightly higher on thiazolidinediones and slightly lower on metformin. Overall, these are reassuring data regarding the safety of these drugs in older patients who have HF. (Nonetheless, metformin retains a black box warning against use in HF requiring pharmacotherapy, and thiazolidinediones are not recommended in New York Heart Association class III or IV status.)

Also unresolved is the potential role of combined PPAR α and γ agonists. Muraglitazar, the first such agent to reach the US Food and Drug Administration (FDA) for consideration of approval, is currently the subject of significant controversy. The drug was recommended for approval by the Endocrinology and Metabolic Drugs division of the FDA, but data relating to the drug were recently reanalyzed by authors not on the committee and published in the *Journal of the American Medical Association*. Both the original article and the accompanying editorial express concerns about an increased RR (2.23) for death, myocardial infarction, or stroke in the group treated with muraglitazar [78,79]. When transient ischemic attack and CHF were included in the outcome measures, the RR increased further (to 2.62) [78]. This issue will not be resolved without further investigation.

Summary

Epidemiologic data clearly demonstrate an association between diabetes and HF. This relationship appears to strengthen in patients hospitalized for HF. The existence of an independent diabetic cardiomyopathy is suggested in many studies. However, because of multiple comorbidities found in the diabetic patient, especially hypertension and ischemic heart disease, it has been hard to demonstrate. A more recent study designed specifically to address the existence of ICM in the diabetic patient does suggest an association [13]. Physiologic studies are more easily able to isolate diabetes from other comorbidities and have offered evidence of diabetic cardiomyopathy by various mechanisms.

In caring for the diabetic patient, one must pay meticulous attention to control of lipids, blood pressure, and glycemia, because all are potentially implicated in this disease. Early screening by BNP or echocardiography should be considered, because

physical evidence of early diabetic cardiomyopathy may be difficult to discern. Early detection of the disease should prompt intensification of risk factor control and use of agents known to affect the course of HF, such as β-blockers and RAS blockers. Early use of insulin sensitizers in the insulin-resistant patient offers protection against metabolic defects associated with diabetes. With careful monitoring, thiazolidinediones may be used in early HF; prospective data regarding their effect on progression to HF are not yet available.

References

[1] Kannel WB, McGee DL. Diabetes and cardiovascular disease: the Framingham study. JAMA 1979; 241:2035–8.

[2] Nichols GA, Hillier TA, Erbey JR, et al. Congestive heart failure in type 2 diabetes: prevalence, incidence, and risk factors. Diabetes Care 2001;24:1614–9.

[3] Aronow WS, Ahn C. Incidence of heart failure in 2737 older persons with and without diabetes mellitus. Chest 1999;115:867–8.

[4] Amato L, Paolisso G, Cacciatore F, et al. Congestive heart failure predicts the development of non-insulin-dependent diabetes mellitus in the elderly: the Osservatorio Geriatrico Regione Campania Group. Diabetes Metab 1997;23:213–8.

[5] Mazza A, Tikhonoff V, Casiglia E, et al. Predictors of congestive heart failure mortality in elderly people from the general population. Int Heart J 2004; 46:419–31.

[6] Reis SE, Holubkov R, Edmundowicz D, et al. Treatment of patients admitted to the hospital with congestive heart failure: specialty-related disparities in practice patterns and outcomes. J Am Coll Cardiol 1997;30:733–8.

[7] Fonarow G. Approach to the management of diabetic patients with heart failure: role of thiazolidinediones. Am Heart J 2004;148:551–8.

[8] Bell DSH, Ovalle F. Frequency of diabetes in patents admitted to the hospital because of congestive heart failure [abstract]. Diabetes 2001;50:A456.

[9] Tenenbaum A, Fisman EZ, Adler Y, et al. Functional class in patients with heart failure is associated with the development of diabetes. Am J Med 2003;114:271–5.

[10] Grundy SM. Higher incidence of new-onset diabetes in patients with heart failure. Am J Med 2003;114: 331–2.

[11] Rubler S, Dlugash J, Yuceoglu YZ, et al. New type of cardiomyopathy associated with diabetic glomerulosclerosis. Am J Cardiol 1972;30:595–602.

[12] Coughlin SS, Pearle DL, Baughman KL, et al. Diabetes mellitus and risk of idiopathic dilated cardiomyopathy. Ann Epidemiol 1994;4:67–74.

[13] Bertoni AG, Kasper EK, Tsai A, et al. Diabetes and

idiopathic cardiomyopathy: a nationwide case-control study. Diabetes Care 2003;26:2791–5.

[14] Sohn DW, Chai IH, Lee DJ, et al. Assessment of mitral annulus velocity by Doppler tissue imaging in the evaluation of left ventricular diastolic function. J Am Coll Cardiol 1997;30:595–602.

[15] Schwannwell CM, Scheppenheim M, Perings S, et al. Left ventricular diastolic dysfunction as an early manifestation of diabetic cardiomyopathy. Cardiology 2002;98:33–9.

[16] Suys B, Katier N, Rooman RPA, et al. Female children and adolescents with type 1 diabetes have more pronounced early echocardiographic signs of diabetic cardiomyopathy. Diabetes Care 2004;27:1947–53.

[17] Nicolino A, Longobardi G, Furgi G, et al. Left ventricular diastolic filling in diabetes mellitus with and without hypertension. Am J Hypertens 1995;8:382–9.

[18] Di Bonito P, Cuomo S, Moio N, et al. Diastolic dysfunction in patients with non–insulin-dependent diabetes mellitus of short duration. Diabet Med 1996; 13:321–4.

[19] Redfield MM, Jacobsen SJ, Burnett Jr JC, et al. Burden of systolic and diastolic dysfunction in the community. JAMA 2003;289:194–202.

[20] Poirier P, Bogaty P, Garneau C, et al. Diastolic dysfunction in normotensive men with well-controlled type 2 diabetes: importance of maneuvers in echocardiographic screening for preclinical diabetic cardiomyopathy. Diabetes Care 2001;24:5–10.

[21] Friedman NE, Levisky LL, Edidin DV, et al. Echocardiographic evidence for impaired myocardial performance in children with type 1 diabetes mellitus. Am J Med 1982;73:846–50.

[22] Mbanya JC, Sobngwi E, Mbanya DS, et al. Left ventricular mass and systolic function in African diabetic patients: association with microalbuminuria. Diabetes Metab 2001;27:378–82.

[23] Fang ZY, Yuda S, Anderson V, et al. Echocardiographic detection of early diabetic myocardial disease. J Am Coll Cardiol 2003;41:611–7.

[24] Iribarren C, Karter AJ, Go AS, et al. Glycemic control and heart failure among adult patients with diabetes. Circulation 2001;103:2668–73.

[25] Shishehbor M, Hoogwerf B, Schoenhagen P, et al. Relation of hemoglobin A_{1c} to left ventricular relaxation in patients with type 1 diabetes mellitus and without overt heart disease. Am J Cardiol 2003; 91:1514–7.

[26] Devereux RB, Roman MJ, Paranicas M, et al. Impact of diabetes on cardiac structure and function: the Strong Heart Study. Circulation 2000;101:2271–6.

[27] Cooper M. Importance of advanced glycation end products in diabetes associated cardiovascular and renal disease. Am J Hypertens 2004;17:31S–8S.

[28] Candido R, Forbes JM, Thomas MC, et al. A breaker of advanced glycation end products attenuates diabetes-induced myocardial structural changes. Circ Res 2003; 92:785–92.

[29] Nunoda S, Genda A, Sugihara N, et al. Quantitative approach to the histopathology of the biopsied right ventricular myocardium in patients with diabetes mellitus. Heart Vessels 1985;1:43–7.

[30] Picano E, Pelosi G, Marzilli M, et al. In vivo quantitative ultrasonic evaluation of myocardial fibrosis in humans. Circulation 1990;81:58–64.

[31] Gonzalez-Vilchez F, Ayuela J, Ares M, et al. Oxidative stress and fibrosis in incipient myocardial dysfunction in type 2 diabetic patients. Int J Cardiol 2003; 101:53–8.

[32] Waczulikova I, Ziegelhoffer A, Orszaghova Z, et al. Fluidising effect of resrcylidene aminoguanidine on sarcolemmal membranes in streptozotocin-diabetic rats: blunted adaptation of diabetic myocardium to Ca overload. J Physiol Pharmacol 2002;53:727–39.

[33] Garcia S, Virag L, Jagtap P, et al. Diabetic endothelial dysfunction: the role of poly (ADP-ribose) polymerase activation. Nat Med 2001;7:108–13.

[34] Szabo C. Roles of poly(ADP-ribose) polymerase activation in the pathogenesis of diabetes mellitus and its complications. Pharmacol Res 2005;52:60–71.

[35] Oliver MF, Opie LH. Effects of glucose and fatty acids on myocardial ischaemia and arrhythmias. Lancet 1994;343:155–8.

[36] Mjos OD. Effect of free fatty acids on myocardial function and oxygen consumption in intact dogs. J Clin Invest 1991;50:1386–9.

[37] Zhou YT, Grayburn P, Karim A, et al. Lipotoxic heart disease in obese rats: implications for human obesity. Proc Natl Acad Sci USA 2000;97(4):1784–9.

[38] Young ME, Laws F, Goodwin GW, et al. Reactivation of peroxisome proliferators–activator receptor α is associated with contractile dysfunction in hypertrophied rat heart. J Biol Chem 2001;276:44390–5.

[39] Finck B, Lehman J, Leone T, et al. The cardiac phenotype induced by PPARα overexpression mimics that caused by diabetes mellitus. J Clin Invest 2002; 109:121–30.

[40] Cooper GJS, Phillips ARJ, Choong SY, et al. Regeneration of the heart in diabetes by selective copper chelation. Diabetes 2004;53:2501–8.

[41] Cooper GJS, Chan YK, Dissanayake AM, et al. Demonstration of a hyperglycemia-driven pathogenic abnormality of copper homeostasis in diabetes and its reversibility by selective chelation. Diabetes 2005; 54:1468–76.

[42] Wakasaki H, Koya D, Schoen F, et al. Targeted overexpression of protein kinase C $B2$ isoform in myocardium causes cardiomyopathy. Proc Natl Acad Sci USA 1997;94:9320–5.

[43] Young ME, McNulty P, Tegtemeyer H. Adaptation and maladaptation of the heart in diabetes: part II, potential mechanisms. Circulation 2002;105:1861–70.

[44] Bristow M. Etomoxir: a new approach to treatment of chronic heart failure. Lancet 2000;356:1621–2.

[45] Genda A, Mizuno S, Nunoda S, et al. Clinical studies on diabetic myocardial disease using exercise testing with myocardial scintigraphy and endomyocardial biopsy. Clin Cardiol 1986;9:375–82.

[46] Sunni S, Bishop SP, Kent SP, et al. Diabetic cardiomyopathy: a morphological study of intramyocardial arteries. Arch Pathol Lab Med 1986;110:375–81.

[47] Yarom R, Zirkin H, Stammler G, et al. Human coronary microvessels in diabetes and ischaemia. Morphometric study of autopsy material. J Pathol 1992; 166(3):265–70.

[48] Yoon Y, Uchida S, Masuo O, et al. Progressive attenuation of myocardial vascular endothelial growth factor expression is a seminal event in diabetic cardiomyopathy. Circulation 2004;111:2073–85.

[49] Vinik AI, Maser RE, Mitchell BD, et al. Diabetic autonomic neuropathy. Diabetes Care 2003;26(5):1553–79.

[50] Maser RE, Lenhard MJ. Cardiovascular autonomic neuropathy due to diabetes mellitus: clinical manifestations, consequences and treatment. J Clin Endocrinol Metab 2005;90(10):5896–903.

[51] Fang ZY, Prins JB, Marwick T. Diabetic cardiomyopathy: evidence, mechanisms and therapeutic implications. Endocr Rev 2004;25(4):543–67.

[52] Kreiner G, Wolzt M, Fasching P, et al. Myocardial M(123-I) iodobenzylguanidine scintigraphy for the assessment of adrenergic cardiac innervation in patients with IDDM. Comparison with cardiovascular reflex tests and relationship to left ventricular function. Diabetes 1995;44:543–9.

[53] Taskiran M, Fritz-Hansen T, Rasmussen V, et al. Decreased myocardial perfusion reserve in diabetic autonomic neuropathy. Diabetes 2002;51:3306–10.

[54] Bristow MR. Why does the myocardium fail? Insights from basic science. Lancet 1998;352(Suppl 1):SI8–14.

[55] Eichhorn EJ, Bristow MR. Medical therapy can improve the biological properties of the chronically failing heart: a new erea in the treatment of hear failure. Circulation 1996;94:2285–96.

[56] McDonagh TA, Morrison CE, Lawrence A, et al. Symptomatic and asymptomatic left-ventricular systolic dysfunction in an urban population. Lancet 1999;350:829–33.

[57] Stone PH, Raabe DS, Jaffe AS, et al. Prognostic significance of location and type of myocardial infarction: independent adverse outcome associated with anterior location. J Am Coll Cardiol 1988;11:453–63.

[58] Levy D, Larson MG, Vasan RS, et al. The progression from hypertension to congestive heart failure. JAMA 1996;275:1557–62.

[59] Hunt SA, Baker DW, Chin MH, et al. ACC/AHA guidelines for the evaluation and management of chronic heart failure in the adult: executive summary. A report of the American College of Cardiology/ American Heart Association Task Force on Practice Guidelines (committee to revise the 1995 Guidelines for the Evaluation and Management of Heart Failure). J Am Coll Cardiol 2001;38:2101–13.

[60] Joint National Committee on Prevention DEaToHBP. The sixth report of the Joint National Committee on Prevention, Detection, Evaluation, and Treatment of High Blood Pressure. Arch Intern Med 1997; 157:2413–46.

[61] Adler AI, Stratton IM, Neil HAW, et al. Association of systolic blood pressure with macrovascular and microvascular complications of type 2 diabetes (UKPDS 36): prospective observational study. BMJ 2000;321:412–9.

[62] Marantz PR, Tobin JN, Wassertheil-Smoller S, et al. The relationship between left ventricular systolic function and congestive heart failure diagnosed by clinical criteria. Circulation 1988;77:607–12.

[63] Bittner V, Weiner DH, Yusuf S, et al. Prediction of mortality and morbidity with a 6-minute walk test in patients with left ventricular dysfunction: SOLVD investigators. JAMA 1993;270:1702–7.

[64] Bourassa MG, Gurne O, Bangdiwala SI, et al. Natural history and patterns of current practice in heart failure: the Studies of Left Ventricular Dysfunction (SOLVD) investigators. J Am Coll Cardiol 1993; 22:14A–9A.

[65] Struthers AD, Morris AD. Screening for and treating left-ventricular abnormalities in diabetes mellitus: a new way of reducing cardiac deaths. Lancet 2002; 359:1430–2.

[66] Lainchbury JG, Redfield MM. Doppler echocardiographic-guided diagnosis and therapy of heart failure. Curr Cardiol Rep 1999;1:55–66.

[67] McKenna K, Smith D, Tormey W, et al. Acute hyperglycaemia causes elevation in plasma atrial natriuretic peptide concentrations in type 1 diabetes mellitus. Diabet Med 2000;17:512–7.

[68] McDonagh TA, Robb SD, Murdoch DR, et al. Biochemical detection of left-ventricular systolic dysfunction. Lancet 1998;351:9–13.

[69] Liu JE, Robbins DC, Palmieri V, et al. Association of microalbuminuria with systolic and diastolic left ventricular dysfunction in type 2 diabetes: the Strong Heart Study. J Am Coll Cardiol 2003;42:2022–8.

[70] Arnold JM, Yusuf S, Young J, et al. Prevention of heart failure in patients in the Heart Outcome Prevention Evaluation (HOPE) study. Circulation 2003; 107:1284–90.

[71] United Kingdom Prospective Diabetes Study (UKPDS) Group Investigators. Tight blood pressure control and risk of macrovascular and microvascular complications in type 2 diabetes: UKPDS 38. BMJ 1998;317:703–13.

[72] United Kingdom Prospective Diabetes Study (UKPDS) Group Investigators. Efficacy of atenolol and captopril in reducing risk of macrovascular and microvascular complications in type 2 diabetes: UKPDS 39. BMJ 1998;317:713–20.

[73] Tang WH, Francis GS, Hoogwerf BJ, et al. Fluid retention after initiation of thiazolidinedione therapy in diabetic patients with established chronic heart failure. J Am Coll Cardiol 2003;41:1394–8.

[74] St. John Sutton M, Rendell M, Dandona P, et al. A comparison of the effects of rosiglitazone and glyburide on cardiovascular function and glycemic control in patients with type 2 diabetes. Diabetes Care 2002; 25:2058–64.

[75] Schneider RL, Shaffer SJ for the Pioglitazone 011

Study Group. Long-term echocardiographic assess-ment in patients with type 2 diabetes mellitus. Circu-lation 2002;106:679–84.

[76] Wang CH, Weisel RD, Liu PP, et al. Glitazones and heart failure: critical appraisal for the clinician. Circulation 2003;107:1350–4.

[77] Masoudi FA, Inzucchi SE, Wang Y, et al. Thiazo-lidinediones, metformin, and outcomes in older pa-tients with diabetes and heart failure: an observational study. Circulation 2005;111:583–90.

[78] Nissen SE, Wolski K, Topol EJ. Effect of muraglitazar on death and major adverse cardiovascular events in patients with type 2 diabetes mellitus. JAMA 2005; 294:2581–6.

[79] Brophy JM. Selling safety-lessons from muraglitazar. JAMA 2005;294:2633–5.

ELSEVIER
SAUNDERS

Heart Failure Clin 2 (2006) 81 – 88

HEART
FAILURE
CLINICS

The Rationale and Indications for Angiotensin Receptor Blockers in Heart Failure

Kevin A. Bybee, MD, Sajal Das, MD, James H. O'Keefe, MD*

Mid America Heart Institute, Kansas City, MO, USA

More than 5 million Americans have congestive heart failure (CHF), and the lifetime incidence of this disorder is now approximately 20%. Angiotensin-converting enzyme (ACE) inhibitors improve outcomes in patients who have CHF. Studies show, however, that at least 10% of patients do not tolerate ACE inhibitors because of cough; and 20% of the population who have reduced left ventricular ejection fraction (LVEF) are not receiving ACE inhibitors [1]. Angiotensin receptor blockers (ARBs) block the angiotensin II receptor and are generally well tolerated. Thus, the ARBs are logical alternatives or adjuncts to ACE inhibitors to counteract the activated renin-angiotensin-aldosterone system (RAAS) and poor prognosis associated with CHF.

Mechanisms of action

Angiotensin II is not only a potent vasoconstrictor, but also a trophic hormone that stimulates growth and hypertrophy of the myocardium and smooth muscle in the wall of blood vessels, leading to adverse structural effects on the heart and vasculature. Additionally, angiotensin II activates other neurohumoral agonists, including aldosterone, norepinephrine, endothelin, and cytokines, leading to potentially deleterious cardiovascular consequences,

such as vasoconstriction, sodium retention, inflammation, atherothrombosis, and atherosclerotic plaque rupture (Fig. 1).

Angiotensin I is converted to angiotensin II by way of the angiotensin-converting enzyme. Alternative pathways are available, however, and provide a mechanism for "ACE escape" during chronic ACE inhibitor therapy. By providing more specific and complete blockade of angiotensin II, ARBs may confer cardiovascular benefits as good as or better than those associated with ACE inhibitors. The concomitant potentiation of bradykinin by ACE inhibitors, but not ARBs, is an additional distinction between the two agents. The up-regulation of bradykinin by ACE inhibition is a double-edged sword. Bradykinin stimulates release of nitric oxide and prostaglandin, likely accounting for some of the benefits noted with ACE inhibitor therapy; however, bradykinin also plays a role in many ACE-inhibitor side effects, such as cough and rash.

Angiotensin receptor blockers shield against consequences of insulin resistance

Approximately 50% of patients who have CHF have diastolic dysfunction without a depressed LVEF [2]. CHF resulting from diastolic dysfunction is typically mediated by chronic hypertensive heart disease with hypertrophy of the arterial smooth muscle wall and left ventricle [2]. The lifetime risk for hypertension for Americans is now 90%, with a progressive increase in prevalence as age increases [3]. The Seventh Report of the Joint National Committee

* Corresponding author. Mid America Heart Institute, 4330 Wornall Road, Suite 2000, Kansas City, MO 64111.
 E-mail address: jhokeefe@cc-pc.com (J.H. O'Keefe).

1551-7136/06/$ – see front matter © 2006 Elsevier Inc. All rights reserved.
doi:10.1016/j.hfc.2005.11.003

heartfailure.theclinics.com

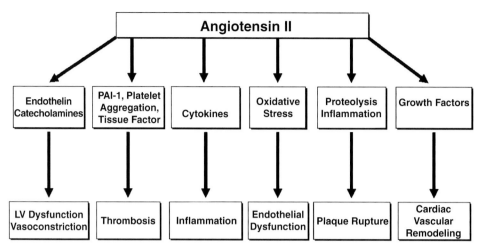

Fig. 1. Adverse cardiovascular effects of angiotensin II. LV, left ventricular; PAI, plasminogen activator inhibitor.

on Prevention, Detection, Evaluation, and Treatment of High Blood Pressure (JNC 7) emphasized the importance of left ventricular hypertrophy as an independent risk factor for cardiovascular disease [4]. Studies show that ARBs improve endothelial function and arterial compliance, and regress left ventricular hypertrophy [5,6]. A meta-analysis including 3767 patients from double-blind, randomized, controlled parallel group trials of equivalent blood-pressure-lowering strategies reported that ARBs regress left ventricular hypertrophy better than ACE inhibitor, calcium channel blockers, diuretics, or beta blockers.

Insulin resistance is both a cause and an effect of CHF [7]. High insulin levels stimulate the cardiac sympathetic nervous system and the angiotensin receptors. A recent trial suggested the link between obesity and subsequent CHF may be mediated by insulin resistance [8,9]. In this trial of 1187 elderly men followed for 9 years, insulin resistance was found to be correlated independently with risk for subsequent CHF development. In the setting of insulin resistance, the cardiovascular system is sensitized to the adverse trophic effects of the RAAS, as evidenced by the frequent development of CHF, diffuse arterial disease, and left ventricular hypertrophy in patients who have diabetes even when the lipid and blood pressure levels are normal [10]. ACE inhibitors and ARBs improve outcomes in patients who have diabetes [11,12] and in those who have insulin-resistant conditions, such as hypertension [13], coronary disease [12], and CHF.

In the Candesartan in CHF: Assessment of Reduction in Mortality and Morbidity (CHARM) trial of

approximately 7601 patients, candesartan reduced development of new diabetes by 22% in patients who had CHF [14]. Recently, a large meta-analysis involving approximately 100,000 randomized patients showed that therapy with an ACE inhibitor or an ARB reduced the incidence of new type 2 diabetes by about 25% [15]. Most of the patients in this meta-analysis had preexisting insulin-resistant conditions, such as hypertension or CHF.

Trials evaluating angiotensin-converting enzyme inhibitors compared with angiotensin receptor blockers in congestive heart failure

Several large, randomized clinical trials evaluating the effectiveness of ARBs in patients who have systolic left ventricular (LV) dysfunction have been performed and published [16–22]. The clinical trials performed to date evaluated the comparative effectiveness of ARBs and ACE inhibitors, and the incremental benefit of adding ARB therapy to ACE inhibitor therapy in patients who have symptomatic LV systolic dysfunction (Table 1). Initial trials of ARBs in patients who have CHF demonstrated that ARBs were able to improve heart failure symptoms and improve neurohormonal and hemodynamic parameters, but lacked the power to assess effects on hard cardiovascular outcomes [23–26]. A recent study showed that valsartan, 80 mg daily, but not enalapril, 5 mg daily, lowered brain natriuretic peptide (BNP) levels and reduced sympathetic nervous system activity in patients who have CHF [27].

Table 1
Randomized trials of angiotensin receptor blockers in chronic heart failure

Trial [Ref. no.]	Study Medications	Population	End-point	Event rates (%)	Absolute/relative risk reduction	NNT	P value
OPTIMAAL [18]	Losartan vs captopril	Post-MI; LVEF <35% or LVH or anterior MI	All-cause mortality	Losartan: 18 Captopril: 16	2%/11.1%	50	.07
VALIANT [19]	Valsartan vs captopril vs captopril/valsartan	Post-MI; LVEF <40%	All-cause mortality	Valsartan: 19.9 Captopril: 19.5 Captopril + valsartan: 19.3	—	—	NS
ELITE II [17]	Losartan vs captopril	CHF; LVEF <40%	Mortality	Losartan: 17.7 Captopril: 15.9	1.8%/10.8%	56	.16
CHARM-Alternative [21]	Candesartan vs placebo	CHF; LVEF <40%	CV mortality/HF hospitalization	Candesartan: 33 Placebo: 40	7%/17.5%	14	<.01
Val-HeFT [20]	Valsartan vs placebo	CHF; LVEF <40%; 93% on ACEI	CV mortality	Valsartan: 19.7 Placebo: 19.4	—	—	NS
			CV mortality and CV morbidity[a]	Valsartan: 28.8 Placebo: 32.1%	3.3%/10.3%	30	.009
CHARM-Added [22]	Candesartan vs placebo	CHF; LVEF <40%; on ACEI	CV mortality/HF hospitalization	Candesartan 38% Placebo 42%	4%/9.5%	25	.01

Abbreviations: CV, cardiovascular; LVH, left ventricular hypertrophy; NNT, number needed to treat.
[a] Hospitalization for HF, cardiac arrest with resuscitation, outpatient intravenous (IV) inotrope or IV vasodilator treatment.

The ELITE trials

The Evaluation of Losartan in the Elderly (ELITE I) trial was a small (n = 722), randomized trial evaluating losartan versus captopril in elderly patients who had CHF [16]. Surprisingly, mortality (a prespecified secondary endpoint) in the patients treated with losartan was reduced by 54% compared with those receiving captopril. The ELITE II trial was performed subsequently to validate the ELITE I findings [17]. ELITE II was a larger randomized clinical trial evaluating losartan and captopril in 3152 patients, aged 60 years and older, who had symptomatic CHF New York Heart Assocation (NYHA) class II to IV and LVEF less than 40%. Patients were followed for a mean 1.5 years with all-cause mortality prespecified as the primary endpoint. Patients randomized to receive losartan were titrated up to a goal dosage of 50 mg daily, whereas the goal dosage in the captopril-treated patients was 50 mg three times daily. In contrast to the ELITE I findings, in elderly patients who had chronic symptomatic heart failure and were treated with losartan, all-cause mortality was not reduced compared with captopril (17.7% versus 15.9%; hazard ratio 1.13, 95% CI, 0.95–1.35; $P = .16$). There was no significant difference in hospitalization rates for CHF or for the combined endpoint of resuscitated cardiac arrests or sudden cardiac deaths. It was noted that patients in the captopril group were significantly more likely to discontinue the drug because of medication-related side effects. Losartan was better tolerated than captopril. This trial was criticized for using low dosages of losartan compared with moderate to high dosages of captopril.

Trials evaluating angiotensin-converting enzyme inhibitors compared with angiotensin receptor blockers in congestive heart failure following acute myocardial infarction

The OPTIMAAL trial

The OPTIMAAL (Optimal Trial in Myocardial Infarction with the Angiotensin II Antagonist Losartan) trial compared the effects of losartan and captopril on mortality and morbidity in post-myocardial infarction (MI) patients who had LVEF less than 35%, end-diastolic dimension greater than 65 mm, left ventricular hypertrophy, or transmural anterior myocardial infarction/new left bundle branch block [18]. The 5477 enrolled patients received losartan (up-titrated to 50 mg daily) or captopril (up-titrated to 50 mg three times daily) and were followed for an average 2.7 years. Patients who had prior ACE inhibitor or ARB use were excluded from the trial. During follow-up, there were 937 total deaths, including 447 in the captopril group and 499 in the losartan group. There was a trend toward improved all-cause mortality in the captopril-treated patients ($P = .069$) with a small, yet statistically significant reduction in cardiovascular mortality (relative risk 1.17; 95% CI, 1.01–1.34, $P = .032$), suggesting that captopril may be superior to losartan in high-risk, post-infarct patients. However, all other analyzed endpoints were similar between the two groups. As in the ELITE II trial, the OPTIMAAL trial used a low dosage of losartan, 50 mg/d, which may have biased the results in favor of the captopril arm.

The VALIANT trial

VALIANT (Valsartan in Acute Myocardial Infarction Trial) randomized post-MI patients who had LV systolic dysfunction to valsartan (160 mg daily), captopril (50 mg three times daily), or the combination of valsartan (80 mg twice daily) and captopril (50 mg three times daily) [19]. The mean baseline ejection fraction was 35%. In total, 50% of patients received reperfusion therapy, either in the form of thrombolysis in 35% or percutaneous coronary intervention in 15%. No differences in mortality or cardiovascular morbidity were observed during the average 25-month follow-up period, suggesting that valsartan is equivalent to captopril in postinfarct patients who have LV systolic dysfunction. The valsartan mortality benefit was 99.6% of that observed in the captopril group. As would be expected, rates of medication-related side effects were significantly greater in those patients randomized to combination valsartan/captopril therapy.

The CHARM trials

The purpose of the Candesartan in CHF: Assessment of Reduction in Mortality and Morbidity trial was to assess the effects of candesartan on mortality and morbidity in heart failure patients [14,21,28]. There were 7601 CHF patients in the CHARM trial who were divided into three smaller sub-studies. The Charm-Alternative trial enrolled patients who had left ventricular dysfunction intolerant to ACE inhibitors. The Charm-Added trial enrolled patients who had left ventricular systolic dysfunction and were already taking ACE inhibitors. Finally, the Charm-Preserved trial studied CHF patients who had preserved left ventricular function. The primary endpoint of the CHARM Trials was all-cause mortality.

Trials evaluating angiotensin receptor blockers in patients who have congestive heart failure and are intolerant to angiotensin-converting enzyme inhibitors

The CHARM-Alternative trial

The CHARM-Alternative trial randomized 2028 patients who were intolerant to prior ACE inhibitor therapy to either candesartan (up-titrated to a goal of 32 mg) or placebo [21]. Enrolled patients had symptomatic CHF with an LVEF less than 40% and were followed for a median 33.7 months. The patients randomized to receive candesartan were significantly less likely to attain the combined primary endpoint of cardiovascular death or CHF-related hospital admission (33% versus 40%; hazard ratio 0.70; *P*<0.0001). Individually, cardiovascular death rates and rates of hospital admission for CHF were significantly lower in the candesartan group. Patients in the candesartan group were more likely to experience worsening renal function, hypotension, or hyperkalemia compared with the control group. In this trial, candesartan significantly reduced the risk for nonfatal MI [29], largely dismissing earlier concerns that ARBs might not be as effective as ACE inhibitors for preventing acute MI [30].

Angioedema is a common cause of ACE inhibitor intolerance. In the CHARM-Alternative trial, patients who had CHF and previous intolerance to an ACE inhibitor were randomized to either candesartan or placebo [21]. In this study, angioedema occurred in one out of 1013 patients treated with candesartan. A total of 39 patients in this trial had a history of angioedema when previously treated with an ACE inhibitor. During the study, only one of these individuals had recurrent angioedema (which was not life-threatening and did not require hospitalization) when treated with candesartan. The authors of the CHARM-Alternative trial concluded: "A history of angioedema or anaphylaxis on an ACE inhibitor should prompt caution, but does not seem to be a contraindication to use of an ARB" [21].

Trials evaluating angiotensin receptor blockers in addition to angiotensin-converting enzyme inhibitors in patients who have chronic congestive heart failure

The Val-HeFT trial

The Valsartan CHF Trial (Val-HeFT) randomized 5010 patients who had persistently symptom-

atic CHF and LVEF less than 40%, and were already on medical CHF therapy (93% on ACE inhibitors, 33% on beta blockers, 67% on digoxin, and 85% on diuretics), to additional therapy with valsartan (up-titrated to 160 mg twice daily) or placebo [20]. Patients were followed for an average of 23 months. There was no difference in mortality rates between the valsartan and placebo groups: 19.7% versus 19.3%, respectively (*P* = .80). However, fewer patients treated with valsartan reached the combined endpoint of mortality or cardiovascular morbidity (relative risk 0.87; *P* = .009), which was driven by a significant 27.5% reduction in hospital admissions for CHF. Additionally, valsartan-treated patients had significant improvements in CHF symptoms, better quality-of-life scores, and a small but significant improvement in LVEF compared with the placebo group. Subgroup analysis revealed that the patients not receiving concomitant beta blocker or ACE inhibitor therapy derived the greatest benefit from valsartan therapy. Further evaluation demonstrated that patients on concomitant beta blocker, ACE inhibitor, and ARB therapy had an almost 42% greater risk for mortality (*P* = .009) and a nonstatistically significant greater risk for the combined mortality and morbidity endpoint.

The CHARM-Added trial

The CHARM-Added trial randomized 2548 patients already on stable ACE inhibitor therapy and who had persistent symptomatic CHF with LVEF less than 40% to candesartan (up-titrated to 32 mg daily) or placebo [7]. Patients who had NYHA class II symptoms were required to have had a recent hospitalization for cardiac reasons. The patients were followed for an average of 41 months. By completion of the study, 64% of the candesartan patients and 68% of the placebo patients were receiving concomitant beta blocker therapy. The candesartan group was significantly less likely to reach the primary endpoint of combined cardiovascular mortality or CHF-related hospital admission (38% versus 42%, hazard ratio 0.85; 95%, CI, 0.75–0.96; *P* = .01). Individually, cardiovascular mortality and CHF-related hospital admission rates were reduced by 17% in the candesartan group. Patients receiving beta blocker, ACE inhibitor, and ARB therapy were not observed to have increased rates of adverse events. In fact, the great incremental benefit of candesartan therapy was seen in those on concurrent beta blocker and ACE inhibitor therapy.

The CHARM-Preserved trial

This trial enrolled 3025 patients who had preserved left ventricular function (LVEF >40%) and
NYHA Class II–IV CHF, randomized them to
candesartan or placebo, and followed them for
36 months [28]. In this trial, candesartan resulted in
a 9% reduction in the primary endpoint of cardiovascular death and CHF hospitalizations of (22%
versus 24%; *P* = .051) [28].

Summary

In summary, the available clinical trial data demonstrated the following:

- Candesartan therapy improves outcomes in patients who have symptomatic LV systolic dysfunction who are intolerant to ACE inhibitor therapy.
- Losartan and captopril seem to have equivalent
efficacy in stable chronic CHF; however, captopril, 150 mg daily, may be slightly superior to
losartan, 50 mg daily, in patients who had a
recent MI, based on the OPTIMAAL trial.
- Losartan added to ACE inhibitor therapy leads
to modest reductions in rates of CHF hospitalization and CHF symptoms without an effect
on mortality.
- Candesartan added to ACE inhibitor therapy
seems to reduce the risk for cardiovascular-related
mortality and rates of hospitalization for CHF.
- Conflicting data exist whereby candesartan
improved mortality and valsartan worsened mortality when ARB therapy was added to a CHF
regimen of beta blocker and ACE inhibitor therapy.
- Adding ARB therapy to ACE inhibitors increases
the risk for side effects, including hypotension,
worsening renal function, and hyperkalemia.
- ARB therapy produces fewer subjective side
effects than ACE inhibitors and, when used,
should be titrated to goal dosages shown to be
effective in clinical trials (Table 2).
- ARB therapy is not contraindicated in patients
who experience angio edema on an ACE inhibitor.
- ARBs appear to improve prognosis following
acute MI as well as ACE inhibitors.

Implications for clinical practice

The available data addressing ARB therapy in
patients who have symptomatic CHF and LV systolic
dysfunction suggest that ARB therapy should be

Table 2
Starting and goal dosages of angiotensin II receptor blockers
shown to be effective in chronic heart failure

Medication	Dosage	
	Starting	Goal
Losartan	12.5 mg/d	50–100 mg/d
Candesartan	4–8 mg/d	32 mg/d
Valsartan	40 mg twice daily	160 mg twice daily

reserved for patients who are intolerant to ACE
inhibitor therapy and should not be used first-line in
place of ACE inhibitors in patients who have CHF
[21]. The addition of ARB therapy to ACE inhibitor
therapy can be considered in patients who have
hospital admissions for CHF in an attempt to reduce
the chances of subsequent admissions [22]. Additionally, adding ARB therapy could be considered in
patients who have persistent CHF symptoms despite
otherwise optimal medical therapy. Persistent hypertension despite a near maximal antihypertensive
regimen (including, for example, ACE inhibitor, beta
blocker, diuretic and calcium channel blocker) is
another logical indication for ARB therapy in a
patient who has CHF [29,31].

Rather than adding an ARB to an ACE inhibitor
for patients who have persistent NYHA class III and
IV symptoms (despite optimal medical therapy), it
may serve these patients better to add an aldosterone
antagonist, such as aldactone or eplerenone, which
has been shown to reduce mortality in this patient
population [29,32]. Additionally, eplerenone has been
shown to be additive to ACE inhibitor therapy for the
regression of left ventricular hypertrophy and proteinuria in hypertensive patients [33]. The combination
of ACE inhibitor, ARB, and aldactone/eplerenone
therapy cannot be recommended at this time and
would likely carry an unacceptable risk for hyperkalemia. Furthermore, the incremental benefits of
adding an ARB to ACE inhibitor therapy in patients
treated with CHF-device therapy (biventricular pacing with or without an implantable cardioverter-
defibrillator) is not known. These recommendations
are consistent with recent consensus CHF guidelines
from the American Heart Association and the
American College of Cardiology [34].

References

[1] Bart BA, Ertl G, Held P, et al. Contemporary management of patients with left ventricular systolic
dysfunction. Results from the Study of Patients
Intolerant of Converting Enzyme Inhibitors (SPICE)
Registry. Eur Heart J 1999;20(16):1182–90.

[2] Redfield MM, Jacobsen SJ, Burnett Jr JC, et al. Burden of systolic and diastolic ventricular dysfunction in the community: appreciating the scope of the heart failure epidemic. JAMA 2003;289(2):194–202.

[3] Vasan RS, Beiser A, Seshadri S, et al. Residual lifetime risk for developing hypertension in middle-aged women and men: The Framingham Heart Study. JAMA 2002;287(8):1003–10.

[4] Chobanian AV, Bakris GL, Black HR, et al. The Seventh Report of the Joint National Committee on Prevention, Detection, Evaluation, and Treatment of High Blood Pressure: the JNC 7 report. JAMA 2003; 289(19):2560–72.

[5] Wassmann S, Hilgers S, Laufs U, et al. Angiotensin II type 1 receptor antagonism improves hypercholesterolemia-associated endothelial dysfunction. Arterioscler Thromb Vasc Biol 2002;22(7):1208–12.

[6] Klingbeil AU, Schneider M, Martus P, et al. A meta-analysis of the effects of treatment on left ventricular mass in essential hypertension. Am J Med 2003; 115(1):41–6.

[7] Doehner W, Rauchhaus M, Ponikowski P, et al. Impaired insulin sensitivity as an independent risk factor for mortality in patients with stable chronic heart failure. J Am Coll Cardiol 2005;46(6):1019–26.

[8] Murphy R. Insulin resistance might link obesity and congestive heart failure. Nat Clin Pract Cardiovasc Med 2005;2(10):497.

[9] Ingelsson E, Sundstrom J, Arnlov J, et al. Insulin resistance and risk of congestive heart failure. JAMA 2005;294(3):334–41.

[10] O'Keefe JH, Wetzel M, Moe RR, et al. Should an angiotensin-converting enzyme inhibitor be standard therapy for patients with atherosclerotic disease? J Am Coll Cardiol 2001;37(1):1–8.

[11] Tatti P, Pahor M, Byington RP, et al. Outcome results of the fosinopril versus amlodipine cardiovascular events randomized trial (FACET) in patients with hypertension and NIDDM. Diabetes Care 1998;21(4): 597–603.

[12] Yusuf S, Sleight P, Pogue J, et al. Effects of an angiotensin-converting-enzyme inhibitor, ramipril, on cardiovascular events in high-risk patients. The Heart Outcomes Prevention Evaluation Study Investigators. N Engl J Med 2000;342(3):145–53.

[13] Dahlof B, Devereux RB, Kjeldsen SE, et al. Cardiovascular morbidity and mortality in the losartan intervention for endpoint reduction in hypertension study (LIFE): a randomised trial against atenolol. Lancet 2002;359(9311):995–1003.

[14] Pfeffer MA, Swedberg K, Granger CB, et al. Effects of candesartan on mortality and morbidity in patients with chronic heart failure: the CHARM-overall programme. Lancet 2003;362(9386):759–66.

[15] Abuissa H, Jones PG, Marso SP, et al. Angiotensin-converting enzyme inhibitors or angiotensin receptor blockers for prevention of type 2 diabetes a meta-analysis of randomized clinical trials. J Am Coll Cardiol 2005;46(5):821–6.

[16] Pitt B, Segal R, Martinez FA, et al. Randomised trial of losartan versus captopril in patients over 65 with heart failure (evaluation of losartan in the elderly study, ELITE). Lancet 1997;349(9054):747–52.

[17] Pitt B, Poole-Wilson PA, Segal R, et al. Effect of losartan compared with captopril on mortality in patients with symptomatic heart failure: randomised trial–the losartan heart failure survival study ELITE II. Lancet 2000;355(9215):1582–7.

[18] Dickstein K, Kjekshus J. Effects of losartan and captopril on mortality and morbidity in high-risk patients after acute myocardial infarction: the OPTIMAAL randomised trial. Optimal trial in myocardial infarction with angiotensin II antagonist losartan. Lancet 2002;360(9335):752–60.

[19] Pfeffer MA, McMurray JJ, Velazquez EJ, et al. Valsartan, captopril, or both in myocardial infarction complicated by heart failure, left ventricular dysfunction, or both. N Engl J Med 2003;349(20):1893–906.

[20] Cohn JN, Tognoni G. A randomized trial of the angiotensin-receptor blocker valsartan in chronic heart failure. N Engl J Med 2001;345(23):1667–75.

[21] Granger CB, McMurray JJ, Yusuf S, et al. Effects of candesartan in patients with chronic heart failure and reduced left-ventricular systolic function intolerant to angiotensin-converting-enzyme inhibitors: the CHARM-alternative trial. Lancet 2003;362(9386): 772–6.

[22] McMurray JJ, Ostergren J, Swedberg K, et al. Effects of candesartan in patients with chronic heart failure and reduced left-ventricular systolic function taking angiotensin-converting-enzyme inhibitors: the CHARM-added trial. Lancet 2003;362(9386):767–71.

[23] Gottlieb SS, Dickstein K, Fleck E, et al. Hemodynamic and neurohormonal effects of the angiotensin II antagonist losartan in patients with congestive heart failure. Circulation 1993;88(4 Pt 1):1602–9.

[24] Mazayev VP, Fomina IG, Kazakov EN, et al. Valsartan in heart failure patients previously untreated with an ACE inhibitor. Int J Cardiol 1998;65(3):239–46.

[25] Riegger GA, Bouzo H, Petr P, et al. Improvement in exercise tolerance and symptoms of congestive heart failure during treatment with candesartan cilexetil. Symptom, Tolerability, Response to Exercise Trial of Candesartan Cilexetil in Heart Failure (STRETCH) Investigators. Circulation 1999;100(22): 2224–30.

[26] Crozier I, Ikram H, Awan N, et al. Losartan in heart failure. Hemodynamic effects and tolerability. Losartan Hemodynamic Study Group. Circulation 1995;91(3): 691–7.

[27] Kasama S, Toyama T, Hatori T, et al. Comparative effects of valsartan with enalapril on cardiac sympathetic nerve activity and plasma brain natriuretic peptide in patients with congestive heart failure. Heart 2005 [Epub].

[28] Yusuf S, Pfeffer MA, Swedberg K, et al. Effects of candesartan in patients with chronic heart failure and preserved left-ventricular ejection fraction: the

CHARM-preserved trial. Lancet 2003;362(9386):
777–81.

[29] Demers C, McMurray JJ, Swedberg K, et al. Impact of
candesartan on nonfatal myocardial infarction and
cardiovascular death in patients with heart failure.
JAMA 2005;294(14):1794–8.

[30] Verma S, Strauss M. Angiotensin receptor blockers and
myocardial infarction. BMJ 2004;329(7477):1248–9.

[31] Lee GS. Retarding the progression of diabetic nephropathy in type 2 diabetes mellitus: focus on hypertension and proteinuria. Ann Acad Med Singapore
2005;34(1):24–30.

[32] Pitt B, Remme W, Zannad F, et al. Eplerenone, a
selective aldosterone blocker, in patients with left
ventricular dysfunction after myocardial infarction.
N Engl J Med 2003;348(14):1309–21.

[33] Pitt B, Reichek N, Willenbrock R, et al. Effects of
eplerenone, enalapril, and eplerenone/enalapril in
patients with essential hypertension and left ventricular
hypertrophy: the 4E-left ventricular hypertrophy study.
Circulation 2003;108(15):1831–8.

[34] Hunt S, et al. ACC/AHA 2005 guideline update for
the diagnosis and management of chronic CHF in the
adult. Available at: http://www.acc.org/clinical/guidelines/
failure/index.pdf. Accessed December 8, 2005.

ELSEVIER
SAUNDERS

Heart Failure Clin 2 (2006) 89 – 99

Beta Blockade in Diabetic Heart Failure

Mary Ann Lukas, MD, FACC*

Cardiovascular Medicine Development Centre, GlaxoSmithKline, Philadelphia, PA, USA

Activation of multiple neurohormonal systems, including the sympathetic nervous system (SNS), is intrinsic in the pathophysiology of heart failure (HF) [1]. According to the "adrenergic hypothesis," increased cardiac adrenergic drive contributes to loss of myocardial reserve and the progression to left ventricular dysfunction that is characteristic of HF [2]. SNS activation is defined primarily by increased catecholamine levels, especially norepinephrine (NE) [3,4]. Plasma NE is an established prognostic factor in HF, with higher levels indicating worse prognosis [5]. The deleterious effects of NE on the heart include dysfunction and death of cardiac myocytes, increased ventricular size and pressures, increased heart rate, and proarrhythmic effects [3].

Three adrenergic receptors are involved in mediating the consequences of SNS activation in patients who have chronic HF: β_1, α_1, and β_2. Dysfunction and death of cardiac myocytes are mediated by both β_1- and α_1-adrenergic receptors [3]. The action of NE on β_1-adrenergic receptors is chiefly responsible for increases in ventricular size and pressure [3]. The proarrhythmic effect of NE in patients who have HF is believed to be mediated primarily through β_2-receptors [6], and increased heart rate results from stimulation of both β_1- and β_2-receptors [3].

Diabetes and insulin resistance have also been shown to contribute to cardiac injury and subsequent activation of the SNS [7]. Diabetes is associated with hyperglycemia, insulin resistance, and increased free fatty acids (FFA), metabolic changes that are associated with biochemical events contributing to

the production of cardiomyopathy [8]. In the insulin-resistant state, the normal insulin-mediated decrease in vascular resistance is blunted because of a reduction in the synthesis of endothelium-dependent nitric oxide [9], whereas insulin activates the SNS, leading to an increase in peripheral vascular resistance and impaired glucose delivery to the skeletal muscle [10,11]. Hyperinsulinemia is associated with increased FFA levels in patients who have diabetes, and activation of the SNS in patients who have diabetes results in increased myocardial use of FFA. Thus, the 'negative' myocardial response to the diabetic environment consists of cardiac myocyte hypertrophy, myocardial ischemia, cardiac arrhythmias, interstitial fibrosis, and intracellular triglyceride accumulation resulting from increased fatty acid uptake [12,13].

Cardiovascular effects of beta blockers

The cardiovascular benefits of beta blockade include the reduction in myocardial wall stress, reversal of cardiovascular remodeling, prevention of arrhythmias, anti-ischemic effects, and antiatherogenic effects [14]. Beta blockers provide an antiarrhythmic effect by reducing sympathetic activity and increasing cardiac vagal tone. The anti-ischemic effects of beta blockers derive from the activities of these agents to decrease heart rate and blood pressure, prolong diastole, increase blood flow through the myocardium, and reduce oxygen consumption [14]. Beta blockers also have antiatherogenic and anti-inflammatory effects that stabilize atheromatous plaque and lower the rate of plaque rupture [15]. The inhibitory effect on atherosclerosis may be caused by mechanisms that help mitigate the disease process, and other factors that reduce arterial wall stress, modify the structure of low-density lipoproteins in a manner that reduces

* GlaxoSmithKline, 200 North 16th Street, FP1380, Philadelphia, PA 19102.
E-mail address: mary.ann.lukas@gsk.com

1551-7136/06/$ – see front matter © 2006 Elsevier Inc. All rights reserved.
doi:10.1016/j.hfc.2005.11.005

their potential to bind to the arterial wall, and increase the synthesis of prostacyclin [14]. Box 1 lists the potential cardiovascular benefits of beta blockade in patients who have diabetes.

Benefits of beta blockade in patients who are diabetic

There is a strong rationale in favor of the use of beta blocker therapy in the patient who is diabetic. The United Kingdom Prospective Diabetes Study demonstrated that beta blockade can prevent HF in the patient who is diabetic [16]. This study was designed to analyze the effects of tight control of blood pressure in patients who have diabetes, and patients who enrolled received either a beta blocker or an angiotensin-converting enzyme (ACE) inhibitor as their main treatment. A 56% reduction in the risk for HF was seen in patients allocated to tight control of blood pressure, with no difference in the risk reduction between the two pharmacologic treatments [16].

Following an acute myocardial infarction (MI), FFA levels are extremely high in the patient who has diabetes [17]. Beta blockade reduces myocardial FFA use by lowering the cardiac workload and oxygen consumption. This major change in myocardial function results in less myocardial ischemia and damage, a lower risk for arrhythmia, and improved myocardial function, which may account for much of the increased cardioprotective role of beta blockers in the post-MI patient who has diabetes [14].

Antiinflammatory effects are important to both the patient who has diabetes and the patient who is insulin-resistant. In insulin-resistant patients, the C-reactive protein level is proportional to the degree of insulin resistance, demonstrating the proinflammatory state of the patients [18]. Beta blockers have been shown to lower the C-reactive protein level by as much as 40% [19].

Noncardiovascular effects of concern with beta blocker use in patients who have diabetes

Historically, the use of beta blockers in diabetes has been controversial, despite their proven benefits. Beta blockade can promote glucose intolerance through impairment of first-phase insulin secretion, decrease in energy expenditure, propensity for weight gain, and diminution of peripheral blood flow with decrease in insulin and glucose delivery to insulin-sensitive tissues (ie, skeletal muscle) [20–23]. A potential adverse effect of β_1-selective blockade in the patient who is diabetic is vasoconstriction caused by unopposed α-activity in the presence of beta blockade, which can worsen peripheral vascular disease in the patient who is diabetic [15,24]. Vasoconstriction also leads to decreased skeletal-muscle microvascular surface area, which results in decreased insulin-mediated glucose entry into the myocyte and worsening insulin resistance.

Hypoglycemia may be more frequent and severe in the patient who is diabetic and using beta blockers because hepatic glucose production is controlled in part by sympathetic β stimulation. Blockade of the receptors needed for this important protective mechanism results in an increased frequency and severity of hypoglycemia [25]. In addition, beta blockade suppresses adrenergic symptoms of hypoglycemia so that sweating and neuroglycemic symptoms are often the only warning signs of hypoglycemia [26].

Metabolic effects of beta blockers

Pharmacologic differences between beta blockers may compound their effects on metabolic parameters. Both nonselective beta blockers, such as propranolol, and β_1-selective blockers, such as atenolol and metoprolol, have been shown to increase insulin resistance and raise serum insulin levels. These beta blockers may also exacerbate the proatherogenic profile of blood lipids, raising triglyceride and lowering high-density lipoprotein levels. The nonselective beta blocker carvedilol has not been associated with these adverse metabolic effects [27], which may be due to the additional blockade of β_2- and α_1-adrenergic receptors.

β_1-Stimulation augments renin-angiotensin system activity by releasing renin from the kidney, and in turn, angiotensin II further enhances SNS outflow. Accordingly, β_1-receptor stimulation can result in decreased glucose utilization, whereas α_1- or β_2-activity can lead to increased peripheral blood flow and enhanced glucose disposal.

Small trials have compared the effects of different beta blockers on metabolic parameters in patients who have hypertension or HF. Jacob and colleagues [20] investigated the effects of metoprolol and carvedilol in hypertensive patients who were not diabetic; they found a significant increase in insulin sensitivity with carvedilol and a significant decrease with metoprolol after 12 weeks of treatment. In a randomized 24-week trial of carvedilol versus atenolol in patients who had diabetes and hypertension, atenolol-treated patients experienced a decrease in insulin sensitivity and an increase in serum insulin, and an elevation in serum triglyceride and decease in high-density lipoprotein levels. The carvedilol-treated group demonstrated an increase in insulin sensitivity and a decline in serum insulin; serum triglycerides fell and high-density lipoprotein levels rose. Atenolol was associated with a 4% increase in hemoglobin A_{1C} (HbA_{1C}) levels compared with a 1.4% decrease with carvedilol [28].

The double-blind Glycemic Effects in Diabetes Mellitus: Carvedilol-Metoprolol Comparison in Hypertensives (GEMINI) trial randomized 1235 patients who had diabetes and hypertension to carvedilol and metoprolol tartrate for 6 months. Insulin sensitivity improved significantly with carvedilol (-9.1%; $P = .004$) but not metoprolol tartrate (-2.0%; $P = .48$). Additionally, HbA_{1C} levels did not change with carvedilol therapy [29].

Two evaluations of the effects of carvedilol on glucose metabolism have been reported in HF patients who have and do not have diabetes. In a placebo-controlled, 23-week trial, Refsgaard and colleagues [30] found that insulin sensitivity derived from intravenous glucose tolerance test data did not change with carvedilol treatment. Ferrua and colleagues [31] studied HF patients who were not diabetic for 9 months and found impaired glucose tolerance and borderline fasting glycemia in most patients at baseline, which did not change after carvedilol treatment. Fasting insulinemia significantly decreased during carvedilol treatment, with a reduction of insulin sensitivity as assessed by the homeostasis model assessment (HOMA) index.

Experience with beta blockers in heart failure and diabetes

The standard of care for all patients who have HF (including those who have diabetes) caused by left ventricular systolic dysfunction regardless of severity or etiology, should include pharmacotherapy with an ACE inhibitor and a beta blocker, unless the patient has a contraindication to their use or cannot tolerate treatment with these agents. The compelling clinical evidence for reduced mortality and reduced hospitalizations in HF patients who receive beta blocker therapy, specifically bisoprolol, long-acting metoprolol, or carvedilol, has resulted in these therapies being recommended as standard therapy for HF in numerous practice guidelines [32,33]. These agents have all been shown to reduce mortality in pivotal large-scale clinical trials.

Effects in subjects with diabetes in major beta blocker heart failure clinical trials

Among the major beta blocker HF clinical trials, approximately 25% to 30% of patients enrolled were diagnosed with diabetes. In an effort to determine if beta blockers are as useful in HF patients who have diabetes as in those who do not have diabetes, the outcomes in the diabetic subgroups in several of the large trials have been analyzed. The effects of beta blockers on mortality in subjects who had and who did not have diabetes in large-scale clinical HF trials are summarized in Table 1 [34–38].

In the Cardiac Insufficiency Bisoprolol Study II (CIBIS-II), 2647 patients who had moderate-to-severe HF [mostly New York Heart Association (NYHA) class III] receiving standard ACE inhibitor and diuretic therapy were randomized to additional treatment with bisoprolol or placebo [35]. Overall, patients treated with bisoprolol had a 34% reduction in mortality and a 32% reduction in the rate of hospital admissions [35]. Among patients who had diabetes treated with bisoprolol, there was a smaller and statistically nonsignificant trend toward reduced mortality [39].

The Metoprolol Controlled-Release Randomized Intervention Trial in Heart Failure (MERIT-HF) investigated the benefit of extended-release metoprolol succinate in 3991 patients who had HF and proved statistically beneficial in the entire HF population [36]. Subgroup analysis showed that metoprolol succinate reduced the risk for hospitalization for HF in patients who have diabetes by 37% (95% CI, 15%–53%) and by 35% in the nondiabetic group (95% CI, 19%–48%). Although there was a trend

Table 1
Effect of beta blockers on mortality in diabetic and nondiabetic heart failure patients

Study [Ref.]	Diabetic patients (%)	β Blocker	HF severity	Target dosage	Decrease in mortality	
					All patients	Diabetic patients
US Carvedilol [34]	29	Carvedilol	Mild/moderate/severe	6.25–25 mg twice daily[a]	65%[b]; $P<.001$	63%; (8%, 85%)
CIBIS-II [35]	12	Bisoprolol[c]	Moderate/severe	10 mg once daily	34%; $P<.0001$	19%; P=NS
MERIT-HF [36]	25	Metoprolol succinate	Mild/moderate	200 mg once daily	34%; P=.0062	18%; P=NS
COPERNICUS [37]	26	Carvedilol	Severe	25 mg twice daily	35%; P=.0014	32%; P=NS

Abbreviations: CIBIS-II, Cardiac Insufficiency Bisoprolol Study II; COPERNICUS, Carvedilol Prospective Randomized Cumulative Survival; MERIT-HF, Metoprolol CR/XL Randomised Intervention Trial in Congestive Heart Failure; NS, not significant.

[a] If patient weighed >85 kg, 50 mg twice daily.
[b] Not a planned end point.
[c] HF is not an approved indication.

toward decreased all-cause mortality in metoprolol-treated patients who had diabetes, it did not reach statistical significance [40].

The efficacy of the nonselective beta blocker bucindolol compared with placebo was evaluated in 2708 patients who had NYHA class III (92%) to IV (8%) HF and left ventricular ejection fraction (LVEF) less than or equal to 35% in the Beta Blocker Evaluation of Survival Trial (BEST) [41]. In contrast to previous mortality studies in HF, no significant differences were observed between the groups with regard to all-cause mortality [41], although a significant decrease in cardiovascular deaths ($P=.04$), hospitalization because of HF ($P<.001$), and progression to death or transplantation ($P=.04$) were seen with bucindolol. In a retrospective analysis of patients who had (36%) and who did not have (64%) diabetes, the presence of diabetes was independently associated with increased mortality in patients who had ischemic cardiomyopathy but not in those who had a nonischemic etiology. Beta blocker therapy was at least as effective in reducing death or HF hospitalizations, total hospitalizations, HF hospitalizations, and MI in patients who had diabetes compared with patients who did not have diabetes [42].

The Carvedilol Prospective Randomized Cumulative Survival Study (COPERNICUS) showed a significant reduction in all-cause mortality with carvedilol use in 2289 patients who had severe chronic HF [37]. Benefit was seen across all patient subgroups evaluated [43,44]. In COPERNICUS, the statistically significant 35% relative risk reduction in all-cause mortality was the same for patients treated with carvedilol who had and who did not have diabetes [45].

Carvedilol treatment was associated with a significant reduction in all-cause mortality in all patients and in the diabetic subgroup in the US Carvedilol Trials, which enrolled 1098 patients who had primarily mild-to-moderate disease [45,46]. Retrospective analysis of the Multicenter Oral Carvedilol Heart Failure Assessment (MOCHA) trial indicated that carvedilol was effective in both patients who had and who did not have diabetes in reduction of mortality and improvement of left ventricle function [47]. Of note, the slope of the dose/mortality relation was significantly steeper in patients who had diabetes ($P=.013$) [46].

In the Carvedilol Or Metoprolol European Trial (COMET), which enrolled 3029 patients who also primarily had mild or moderate HF and followed them for a mean of 5.5 years, there was an overall 17% survival benefit with carvedilol versus metoprolol tartrate. This benefit persisted in the diabetic subpopulation (relative risk = 15% in the 24% of patients who had baseline diabetes) [48].

The Carvedilol Post-Infarct Survival Control in Left Ventricular Dysfunction (CAPRICORN) trial demonstrated a 29% risk reduction ($P=.002$) in the combined endpoint of all-cause mortality or non-fatal MI with the use of carvedilol versus placebo in 1959 post-MI patients who had left ventricular systolic dysfunction [49]. Subgroup analysis revealed that CAPRICORN patients who had diabetes benefited to the same degree as the subjects overall, with a 26% reduction in the risk for all-cause mortality or nonfatal MI ($P=.013$) [50].

The Study of the Effects of Nebivolol Intervention on Outcomes and Rehospitalisation in Seniors with Heart Failure (SENIORS) assessed the effects of the beta blocker nebivolol versus placebo in 2128 HF patients aged 70 years or older, regardless of ejection fraction (EF). The mean age of patients was 76 years and the mean EF was 36% (35% of patients had an EF of >35%). The primary outcome, a composite of all-cause mortality or cardiovascular hospital admission, was decreased by 14% (95% CI, 74%–99%; $P = .039$) with nebivolol versus placebo. The patients who did not have diabetes appeared to benefit from nebivolol, with a 23% decrease in the primary outcome. The diabetic subgroup (approximately 25% of all patients) had a 5% increase in the primary outcome with nebivolol treatment, although it was not statistically significant (Fig. 1) [51].

Meta-analyses of diabetic subjects in heart failure trials

Because no specific trial has evaluated the effect of beta blocker therapy in patients who have diabetes and HF, recent meta-analyses have been performed to evaluate further if these patients might benefit from beta blocker therapy as much as patients who do not have diabetes. Analyses that combined outcomes from the subpopulation of patients who had diabetes included in many large-scale beta blocker trials concluded that, although beta blockers reduce mortality in HF patients who have diabetes, the reduction may not be as great as that seen in patients who do not have diabetes [52–55].

In the meta-analysis by Shekelle and colleagues [54], which included 8927 patients of whom 21% were identified as diabetic at enrollment, beta blocker use in patients who had diabetes was associated with a 23% mortality reduction compared with a 35%

mortality reduction in patients who did not have diabetes. Although the difference between these risk reductions was not statistically significant, it seems that patients who have diabetes might not benefit to the same degree as patients who do not have diabetes.

Haas and colleagues [53] performed a meta-analysis of 13,129 randomized patients from six HF trials that evaluated bisoprolol, bucindolol, carvedilol, or metoprolol. An average of 25% of patients in each trial had diabetes. The results of this analysis showed an increase in mortality among patients who had diabetes compared with patients who did not have diabetes. The relative risk reduction in mortality in patients who had diabetes and HF on beta blocker treatment versus placebo was 16% (95% CI, 4%–27%; $P = .011$). The relative risk reduction in HF patients who did not have diabetes was 28% (95% CI, 21%–35%; $P < .001$). The difference in the relative risk reductions between subjects who had and subjects who did not have diabetes was of borderline significance ($P = .051$).

These two meta-analyses included trials that used several different beta blockers, each of which have differing pharmacologic actions and resultant effects on cardiovascular and metabolic parameters [20,53,56]. Although these analyses indicated less benefit in the diabetic subgroup with the use of beta blockers, the difference appeared to be less in the large-scale trials with carvedilol; and the results seemed to be driven by the selective beta blockers (Fig. 2) [54,55].

Bisoprolol and metoprolol block the effects of elevated NE levels at the β_1-receptors, which are also down-regulated in chronic HF. Carvedilol also blocks

	Number of Patients Nebivolol/ Placebo	Number of events (rate*) Nebivolol/ Placebo		P value**
All	1067 / 1061	332 (20.3) / 375 (23.9)		
Diabetes				
Not Present	780 / 793	217 (17.4) / 267 (22.5)		0.13
Present	287 / 268	115 (29.3) / 108 (28.3)		

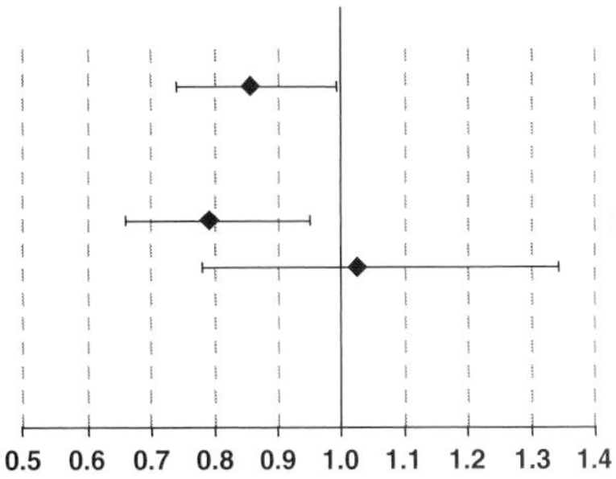

0.5 0.6 0.7 0.8 0.9 1.0 1.1 1.2 1.3 1.4

* Number of events per 100 patient-years of follow-up at risk

** *P* value for interaction: age and ejection fraction considered as continuous variables

Fig. 1. Hazard ratios and 95% confidence intervals for overall, diabetes, and nondiabetes for all-cause death in the SENIORS trial of nebivolol compared with placebo. ◆, hazard ratio. *P*, statistical probability; SENIORS, Study of the Effects of Nebivolol Intervention on Outcomes and Rehospitalisation in Seniors with Heart Failure.

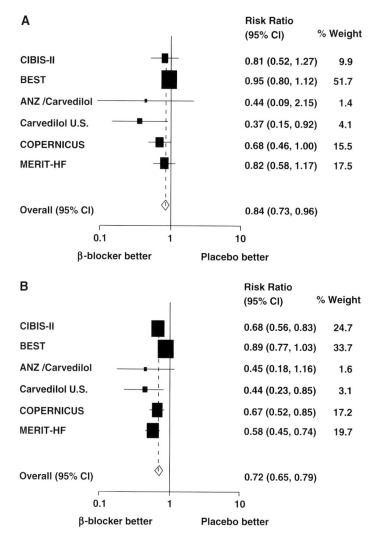

Fig. 2. (*A*) Mantel-Haenszel relative risks (fixed effects) of beta blocker versus placebo for all patients enrolled in trials included in the meta-analysis of Haas and colleagues [52]. Point estimates and 95% confidence intervals (CIs) displayed by box plot. (*B*) Mantel- Haenszel relative risks (fixed effects) of all-cause mortality for patients who had versus patients who did not have diabetes with heart failure. Point estimates and 95% CIs displayed by box plot. ANZ/carvedilol, Australia-New Zealand carvedilol heart failure trial; BEST, Beta Blocker Evaluation of Survival Trial; CIBIS-II, Cardiac Insufficiency Bisoprolol Study II; COPERNICUS, Carvedilol Prospective Randomized Cumulative Survival; MERIT-HF, Metoprolol CR/XL Randomised Intervention Trial in Congestive Heart Failure.

myocardial sympathetic stimulation through the β_2-receptors (which comprise a greater proportion of β-adrenergic receptors in chronic HF) and α-receptors. Furthermore, carvedilol does not reverse the down-regulation of myocardial β_1-receptors as do bisoprolol and metoprolol, which makes fewer receptors available for injurious sympathetic stimulation [57]. Diabetes itself is also associated with significant down-regulation of β_1-myocardial receptors and increased β_2-receptor expression, so that hyperglycemia

is associated with myocardial remodeling [58]. These changes in adrenergic receptor expression might make bisoprolol or metoprolol less effective, and carvedilol more effective, in blunting NE-induced cardiotoxicity in HF patients who have diabetes.

This theory is supported by a meta-analysis of all large-scale carvedilol HF trials. Unlike the previous meta-analyses, which included β_1-selective blockers, this analysis was designed to determine if carvedilol would be as effective in HF patients who were dia-

A

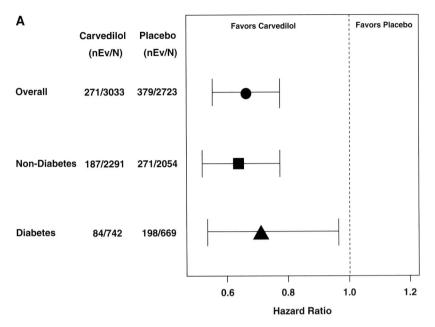

Fig. 3. (*A*) Meta-analysis of carvedilol placebo-controlled heart failure (HF) trials. Hazard ratios and 95% confidence intervals (CIs) for overall (●), diabetes (▲), and nondiabetes (■) for all-cause death. nEv, number of events. (*B*) Meta-analysis of carvedilol placebo-controlled HF trials. Hazard ratios and 95% CIs for all randomized patients (●) in each study, and the diabetic (▲) and nondiabetic (■) subgroups within each study. Estimates from trials with small number of events may not be precise. ANZ, Australia-New Zealand trial; CAPRICORN, Carvedilol Post-Infarct Survival Control in Left Ventricular Dysfunction trial; CARV, carvedilol heart failure trials program; COPERNICUS, Carvedilol Prospective Randomized Cumulative Survival; Diab, diabetic; mHF, mild HF; MOCHA, Multicenter Oral Carvedilol Heart Failure Assessment; nEv, number of events; Non, nondiabetic; PRECISE, Prospective Randomized Evaluation of Carvedilol on Symptoms and Exercise; sHF, severe HF. (*From* Bell DSH, Lukas MA, Holdbrook FK, Fowler MB. The effect of carvedilol on mortality risk in heart failure patients with diabetes: results of a meta-analysis. Curr Med Res Opin 2006;22(2):287–96; with permission.)

betic as in those who were not diabetic. The analysis demonstrated that carvedilol does provide the same survival benefit in patients who have HF and diabetes as it does in HF patients who do not have diabetes. All-cause mortality was significantly reduced in both patients who have diabetes (RR = 28%; CI 3%, 46%; *P* = .029) and patients who did not have diabetes (RR = 37%; CI 22%, 48%; *P* < .0001) with carvedilol therapy versus placebo (Fig. 3A and B).

Safety

Numerous clinical trials and open label studies have demonstrated that beta blockers, when used appropriately, are generally well-tolerated in patients who have HF. Concerns exist about potential adverse events in HF patients treated with beta blockers, however, particularly if the patients have concomitant diabetes [59]. Fewer data are available on the safety profile of beta blockade in patients who have HF and diabetes. In MERIT-HF, the discontinuation rates because of adverse events were higher for patients who had diabetes and were on placebo than for patients who had diabetes and were on metoprolol succinate. In the diabetic group, 31 patients on placebo discontinued the study drug because of HF compared with 18 in the metoprolol group Adverse events were more often reported in the diabetic group than in the nondiabetic group, but regardless of diabetic status, were more often reported with placebo than metoprolol. The most frequent adverse events reported in the diabetic group were worsening HF and hyperglycemia, and these were similar in the metoprolol-treated and placebo-treated groups [55]. In patients who were diabetic and were treated with bisoprolol in the CIBIS-II trial, the number of permanent withdrawals was slightly lower in patients treated with bisoprolol versus placebo [39].

The tolerability of carvedilol was assessed in a retrospective population analysis of over 800 patients with mild-to-severe HF that included patients with "traditional" precautions in the Carvedilol Open Label Assessment study (COLA). In this study,

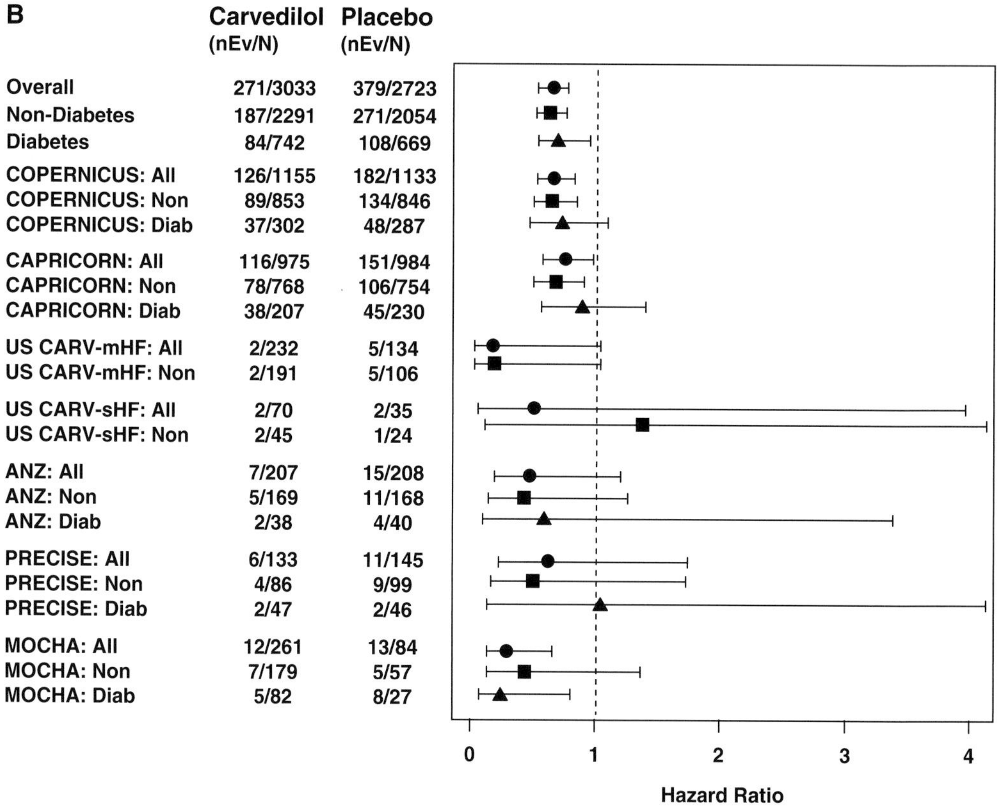

B

	Carvedilol (nEv/N)	Placebo (nEv/N)
Overall	271/3033	379/2723
Non-Diabetes	187/2291	271/2054
Diabetes	84/742	108/669
COPERNICUS: All	126/1155	182/1133
COPERNICUS: Non	89/853	134/846
COPERNICUS: Diab	37/302	48/287
CAPRICORN: All	116/975	151/984
CAPRICORN: Non	78/768	106/754
CAPRICORN: Diab	38/207	45/230
US CARV-mHF: All	2/232	5/134
US CARV-mHF: Non	2/191	5/106
US CARV-sHF: All	2/70	2/35
US CARV-sHF: Non	2/45	1/24
ANZ: All	7/207	15/208
ANZ: Non	5/169	11/168
ANZ: Diab	2/38	4/40
PRECISE: All	6/133	11/145
PRECISE: Non	4/86	9/99
PRECISE: Diab	2/47	2/46
MOCHA: All	12/261	13/84
MOCHA: Non	7/179	5/57
MOCHA: Diab	5/82	8/27

Hazard Ratio (scale 0 1 2 3 4)

Fig. 3 (*continued*).

88% of all patients tolerated (defined as maintaining treatment for 3 months or more after initiation) treatment with carvedilol (mean dose: 42 mg twice daily). Of patients who had diabetes, 86% tolerated carvedilol, a similar rate as the entire population. The two most common reasons for discontinuation of carvedilol were worsening HF and symptomatic hypotension. This study showed that the tolerability of carvedilol was high in HF patients who had diabetes, in practice, outside of the controlled clinical-study setting [60]. In the recently reported COLA-II, 1030 patients who had HF and who were more than 70 years of age were similarly assessed; approximately 30% of the population had diabetes. The presence of diabetes did not affect tolerability; in fact, the presence of diabetes was a predictor of good tolerability [61].

The efficacy and tolerability of carvedilol was also assessed in a smaller trial of 193 HF patients who had and who did not have diabetes. Carvedilol therapy for 12 months resulted in a significant increase in LVEF and improvement in NYHA functional class. This improvement was comparable in patients who had and who did not have diabetes. No significant difference in adverse event incidence was noted between the patients who had and who did not have diabetes. A high degree of tolerability was observed with long-term administration of carvedilol in HF patients who had diabetes in this small trial [62].

Summary

The epidemiologic overlap between type 2 diabetes and HF suggests underlying etiologic links and possible opportunities for synergy in therapeutic interventions. To date, no randomized clinical trial has investigated beta blocker therapy prospectively in a population of patients who have diabetes and HF. However, the pathophysiologic effects of diabetes on the heart occur, in part, through activation of the SNS. The question of the efficacy of beta blockers in patients who have diabetes and HF and the concern over adverse metabolic effects has limited the use of these agents in this patient population. Clinical trial evidence and recent meta-analysis data confirm the

efficacy of specific beta blockers in patients who
have HF and diabetes. In addition, negative metabolic effects have not been seen with the use of the
nonselective agent carvedilol. Therefore, in the
absence of contraindications, beta blockade should
not be withheld in treating patients who have diabetes
and HF; and their use may be instrumental in
preventing further progression of HF and death in
this population.

References

[1] Eichhorn EJ, Bristow MR. Medical therapy can improve the biological properties of the chronically failing heart. A new era in the treatment of heart failure. Circulation 1996;94:2285–96.

[2] Bristow MR. Mechanism of action of beta-blocking agents in heart failure. Am J Cardiol 1997;80:26L–40L.

[3] Packer M. Beta-adrenergic blockade in chronic heart failure: principles, progress, and practice. Prog Cardiovasc Dis 1998;41:39–52.

[4] Francis GS, Goldsmith SR, Levine TB, et al. The neurohumoral axis in congestive heart failure. Ann Intern Med 1984;101:370–7.

[5] Cohn JN, Levine TB, Olivari MT, et al. Plasma norepinephrine as a guide to prognosis in patients with chronic congestive heart failure. N Engl J Med 1984; 311:819–23.

[6] Billman GE, Castillo LC, Hensley J, et al. Beta 2-adrenergic receptor antagonists protect against ventricular fibrillation: in vivo and in vitro evidence for enhanced sensitivity to beta 2-adrenergic stimulation in animals susceptible to sudden death. Circulation 1997; 96:1914–22.

[7] Dzau V, Braunwald E. Resolved and unresolved issues in the prevention and treatment of coronary artery disease: a workshop consensus statement. Am Heart J 1991;121:1244–63.

[8] Giles TD, Sander GE. Diabetes mellitus and heart failure: basic mechanisms, clinical features, and therapeutic considerations. Cardiol Clin 2004;22:553–68.

[9] Baron AD. The coupling of glucose metabolism and perfusion in human skeletal muscle. The potential role of endothelium-derived nitric oxide. Diabetes 1996; 45(Suppl 1):S105–9.

[10] Egan BM. Insulin resistance and the sympathetic nervous system. Curr Hypertens Rep 2003;5:247–54.

[11] Esler M, Kaye D. Increased sympathetic nervous system activity and its therapeutic reduction in arterial hypertension, portal hypertension and heart failure. Journal of the Autonomic Nervous System 1998;72: 210–9.

[12] Taegtmeyer H, McNulty P, Young ME. Adaptation and maladaptation of the heart in diabetes: part I: general concepts. Circulation 2002;105:1727–33.

[13] Malmberg K, Ryden L, Hamsten A, et al. Effects of insulin treatment on cause-specific one-year mortality and morbidity in diabetic patients with acute myocardial infarction. Diabetes Insulin-Glucose in Acute Myocardial Infarction (DIGAMI) Study Group. Eur Heart J 1996;17:1337–44.

[14] Tse WY, Kendall M. Is there a role for beta-blockers in hypertensive diabetic patients? Diabet Med 1994;11: 137–44.

[15] Bell DS. Use of beta blockers in the patient with diabetes. Endocrinologist 2003;13:116–23.

[16] UK Prospective Diabetes Study Group. Tight blood pressure control and risk of macrovascular and microvascular complications in type 2 diabetes: UKPDS 38. BMJ 1998;317:703–13.

[17] Malmberg K. Prospective randomised study of intensive insulin treatment on long term survival after acute myocardial infarction in patients with diabetes mellitus. Diabetes Mellitus, Insulin Glucose Infusion in Acute Myocardial Infarction (DIGAMI) Study Group. BMJ 1997;314:1512–5.

[18] Frohlich M, Imhof A, Berg G, et al. Association between C-reactive protein and features of the metabolic syndrome: a population-based study. Diabetes Care 2000;23:1835–9.

[19] Jenkins NP, Keevil BG, Hutchinson IV, et al. Beta-blockers are associated with lower C-reactive protein concentrations in patients with coronary artery disease. Am J Med 2002;112:269–74.

[20] Jacob S, Rett K, Wicklmayr M, et al. Differential effect of chronic treatment with two beta-blocking agents on insulin sensitivity: the carvedilol-metoprolol study. J Hypertens 1996;14:489–94.

[21] Jacob S, Rett K, Henriksen EJ. Antihypertensive therapy and insulin sensitivity: do we have to redefine the role of beta-blocking agents? Am J Hypertens 1998;11:1258–65.

[22] Jacob S, Balletshofer B, Henriksen EJ, et al. Beta-blocking agents in patients with insulin resistance: effects of vasodilating beta-blockers. Blood Press 1999;8:261–8.

[23] Sharma AM, Pischon T, Hardt S, et al. Hypothesis: beta-adrenergic receptor blockers and weight gain: a systematic analysis. Hypertension 2001;37:250–4.

[24] Roberts DH, Tsao Y, McLoughlin GA, et al. Placebo-controlled comparison of captopril, atenolol, labetalol, and pindolol in hypertension complicated by intermittent claudication. Lancet 1987;2:650–3.

[25] Popp DA, Tse TF, Shah SD, et al. Oral propranolol and metoprolol both impair glucose recovery from insulin-induced hypoglycemia in insulin-dependent diabetes mellitus. Diabetes Care 1984;7:243–7.

[26] Kerr D, MacDonald IA, Heller SR, et al. Beta-adrenoceptor blockade and hypoglycaemia. A randomised, double-blind, placebo controlled comparison of metoprolol CR, atenolol and propranolol LA in normal subjects. Br J Clin Pharmacol 1990;29:685–93.

[27] Hauf-Zachariou U, Widmann L, Zulsdorf B, et al. A double-blind comparison of the effects of carvedilol and captopril on serum lipid concentrations in patients

with mild to moderate essential hypertension and dyslipidaemia. Eur J Clin Pharmacol 1993;45:95–100.

[28] Giugliano D, Acampora R, Marfella R, et al. Metabolic and cardiovascular effects of carvedilol and atenolol in non-insulin-dependent diabetes mellitus and hypertension. A randomized, controlled trial. Ann Intern Med 1997;126:955–9.

[29] Bakris GL, Fonseca V, Katholi RE, et al. Metabolic effects of carvedilol vs metoprolol in patients with type 2 diabetes mellitus and hypertension: a randomized controlled trial. JAMA 2004;292:2227–36.

[30] Refsgaard J, Thomsen C, Andreasen F, et al. Carvedilol does not alter the insulin sensitivity in patients with congestive heart failure. Eur J Heart Fail 2002; 4:445–53.

[31] Ferrua S, Bobbio M, Catalano E, et al. Does carvedilol impair insulin sensitivity in heart failure patients without diabetes? J Card Fail 2005;11:590–4.

[32] Hunt SA, Abraham WT, Chin MH, et al. ACC/AHA 2005 guideline update for the diagnosis and management of chronic heart failure in the adult: a report of the American College of Cardiology/American Heart Association Task Force on Practice Guidelines (Writing Committee to Update the 2001 Guidelines for the Evaluation and Management of Heart Failure). Circulation 2005;112:e154–235.

[33] Heart Failure Society of America. HFSA guidelines for management of patients with heart failure caused by left ventricular systolic dysfunction—pharmacological approaches. Pharmacotherapy 2000;20:495–522.

[34] Packer M, Bristow MR, Cohn JN, et al. The effect of carvedilol on morbidity and mortality in patients with chronic heart failure. US Carvedilol Heart Failure Study Group. N Engl J Med 1996;334:1349–55.

[35] CIBIS-II Investigators. The Cardiac Insufficiency Bisoprolol Study II (CIBIS-II): a randomised trial. Lancet 1999;353:9–13.

[36] MERIT-HF Investigators. Effect of metoprolol CR/XL in chronic heart failure: Metoprolol CR/XL Randomised Intervention Trial in Congestive Heart Failure (MERIT-HF). Lancet 1999;353:2001–7.

[37] Packer M, Coats AJS, Fowler MB, et al. Effect of carvedilol on survival in severe chronic heart failure. N Engl J Med 2001;344:1651–8.

[38] Australia/New Zealand Heart Failure Research Collaborative Group. Randomised, placebo-controlled trial of carvedilol in patients with congestive heart failure due to ischaemic heart disease. Lancet 1997;349: 375–80.

[39] Erdmann E, Lechat P, Verkenne P, et al. Results from post-hoc analyses of the CIBIS II trial: effect of bisoprolol in high-risk patient groups with chronic heart failure. Eur J Heart Fail 2001;3:469–79.

[40] Wedel H, DeMets D, Deedwania P, et al. Challenges of subgroup analyses in multinational clinical trials: Experiences from the MERIT-HF trial. Am Heart J 2001;142:502–11.

[41] Beta-Blocker Evaluation of Survival Trial Investigators. A trial of the beta-blocker bucindolol in patients with advanced chronic heart failure. N Engl J Med 2001;344:1659–67.

[42] Domanski M, Krause-Steinrauf H, Deedwania P, et al. The effect of diabetes on outcomes of patients with advanced heart failure in the BEST trial. J Am Coll Cardiol 2003;42:914–22.

[43] Krum H, Roecker EB, Mohacsi P, et al. Efficacy and safety of initiating carvedilol in patients with severe chronic heart failure: results of COPERNICUS study. Presented at American Heart Association 75th Scientific Sessions. Chicago, Illinois, November 17–20, 2002. Circulation 2002;106:II612.

[44] Fonarow GC. The role of in-hospital initiation of cardioprotective therapies to improve treatment rates and clinical outcomes. Rev Cardiovasc Med 2002; 3(Suppl 3):S2–10.

[45] Mohacsi P, Fowler MB, Krum H, et al. Should physicians avoid the use of beta-blockers in patients with heart failure who have diabetes? Results of the COPERNICUS study. Presented at the American Heart Association 74th Annual Scientific Sessions [abstract no. 3551]. Anaheim, California, November 14, 2001. Circulation 2001;104(Suppl II):II754.

[46] Bristow MR. Effect of carvedilol on LV function and mortality in diabetic vs non-diabetic patients with ischemic or nonischemic dilated cardiomyopathy. Presented at the American Heart Association 69th Scientific Sessions. New Orleans, Louisiana, November 10–13, 1996. Circulation 1996;84:I644.

[47] Bristow MR, Gilbert EM, Abraham WT, et al. Carvedilol produces dose-related improvements in left ventricular function and survival in subjects with chronic heart failure. MOCHA Investigators. Circulation 1996;94:2807–16.

[48] Poole-Wilson PA, Swedberg K, Cleland JG, et al. Comparison of carvedilol and metoprolol on clinical outcomes in patients with chronic heart failure in the Carvedilol or Metoprolol European Trial (COMET): randomised controlled trial. Lancet 2003;362:7–13.

[49] Investigators CAPRICORN. Effect of carvedilol on outcome after myocardial infarction in patients with left-ventricular dysfunction: the CAPRICORN randomised trial. Lancet 2001;357:1385–90.

[50] Data on file. Philadelphia: GlaxoSmithKline.

[51] Flather MD, Shibata MC, Coats AJ, et al. Randomized trial to determine the effect of nebivolol on mortality and cardiovascular hospital admission in elderly patients with heart failure (SENIORS). Eur Heart J 2005;26:215–25.

[52] Bobbio M, Ferrua S, Opasich C, et al. Survival and hospitalization in heart failure patients with or without diabetes treated with beta-blockers. J Card Fail 2003; 9:192–202.

[53] Haas SJ, Vos T, Gilbert RE, et al. Are beta-blockers as efficacious in patients with diabetes mellitus as in patients without diabetes mellitus who have chronic heart failure? A meta-analysis of large-scale clinical trials. Am Heart J 2003;146:848–53.

[54] Shekelle PG, Rich MW, Morton SC, et al. Efficacy of

angiotensin-converting enzyme inhibitors and beta-blockers in the management of left ventricular systolic dysfunction according to race, gender, and diabetic status. A meta-analysis of major clinical trials. J Am Coll Cardiol 2003;41:1529–38.

[55] Deedwania PC, Giles TD, Klibaner M, et al. Efficacy, safety and tolerability of metoprolol CR/XL in patients with diabetes and chronic heart faiiure: experiences from MERIT-HF. Am Heart J 2005;149:159–67.

[56] Gilbert EM, Abraham WT, Olsen S, et al. Comparative hemodynamic, left ventricular functional, and anti-adrenergic effects of chronic treatment with metoprolol versus carvedilol in the failing heart. Circulation 1996; 94:2817–25.

[57] Yoshikawa T, Port JD, Asano K, et al. Cardiac adrenergic receptor effects of carvedilol. Eur Heart J 1996;17(Suppl B):8–16.

[58] Dincer UD, Bidasee KR, Guner S, et al. The effect of diabetes on expression of beta1-, beta2-, and beta3-adrenoreceptors in rat hearts. Diabetes 2001;50: 455–61.

[59] Krum H. Tolerability of carvedilol in heart failure: clinical trials experience. Am J Cardiol 2004;93:58–63.

[60] Krum H, Ninio D, MacDonald P. Baseline predictors of tolerability to carvedilol in patients with chronic heart failure. Heart 2000;84:615–9.

[61] Krum H, Hill J, Fruhwald F, et al. Tolerability of beta-blockers in elderly patients with chronic heart failure: The COLA II study. Eur J Heart Fail 2005.

[62] Nodari S, Metra M, Dei CA, et al. Efficacy and tolerability of the long-term administration of carvedilol in patients with chronic heart failure with and without concomitant diabetes mellitus. Eur J Heart Fail 2003;5:803–9.

[63] Pepine CJ. Potential role of angiotensin-converting enzyme inhibition in myocardial ischemia and current clinical trials. Clin Cardiol 1997;20:II58–64.

[64] Edwin JK, Garrison JC. Renin and angiotensin. In: Hardman JG, Limbird LE, Molinoff PB, et al, editors. Goodman and Gilman's The Pharmacological Basis of Therapeutics. 9th edition. New York: McGraw-Hill; 1996.

Index

Note: Page numbers of article titles are in **boldface** type.

1551-7136/06/$ – see front matter © 2006 Elsevier Inc. All rights reserved.
doi:10.1016/S1551-7136(06)00029-8

Changing Your Address?

Make sure your subscription changes too! When you notify us of your new address, you can help make our job easier by including an exact copy of your Clinics label number with your old address (see illustration below.) This number identifies you to our computer system and will speed the processing of your address change. Please be sure this label number accompanies your old address and your corrected address—you can send an old Clinics label with your number on it or just copy it exactly and send it to the address listed below.

We appreciate your help in our attempt to give you continuous coverage. Thank you.

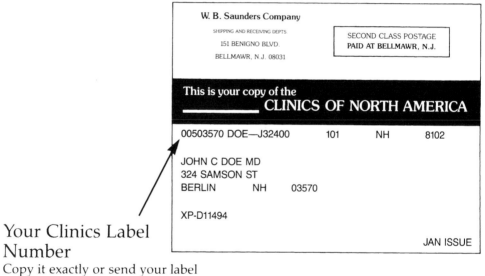

W. B. Saunders Company

SHIPPING AND RECEIVING DEPTS

151 BENIGNO BLVD.

BELLMAWR, N.J. 08031

SECOND CLASS POSTAGE
PAID AT BELLMAWR, N.J.

This is your copy of the
_____ CLINICS OF NORTH AMERICA

00503570 DOE—J32400   101   NH   8102

JOHN C DOE MD
324 SAMSON ST
BERLIN   NH   03570

XP-D11494

JAN ISSUE

Your Clinics Label Number
Copy it exactly or send your label along with your address to:
W.B. Saunders Company, Customer Service
Orlando, FL 32887-4800
Call Toll Free 1-800-654-2452

Please allow four to six weeks for delivery of new subscriptions and for processing address changes.